Health in the Inner City

Edited by
ALISON E. WHILE

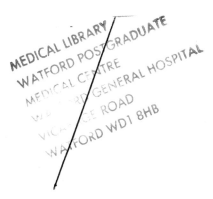

Heinemann Medical Books

Heinemann Medical Books
An imprint of Heinemann Professional Publishing Ltd
Halley Court, Jordan Hill, Oxford OX2 8EJ

OXFORD LONDON SINGAPORE NAIROBI
IBADAN KINGSTON

First published 1989

British Library Cataloguing in Publication Data
Health in the inner city.
   1.   Great Britain. Cities. Inner areas. Man. Health
   I. While, Alison
   613'.0941

ISBN 0-433-18740-9

ISBN 0-433-00152-6

Typeset by Latimer Trend & Company Ltd, Plymouth
Printed in Great Britain by Biddles Ltd
Guildford and Kings Lynn.

Contents

Contributors

Julia Brooking BSc PhD RMN SRN Cert Ed
Senior Lecturer in Psychiatric Nursing
Institute of Psychiatry and Bethlem Royal and Maudsley Hospital University of London, De Crespigny Park, London, SE5 8AF

Gillian Chapman BSc MSc PhD SRN RSCN
Formerly Lecturer
Department of Nursing Studies, King's College, University of London, 552 King's Road, London, SW10 0UA.

Julian Hillman BA MA BPhil/CQSW
Area Social Services Officer
London Borough of Hammersmith and Fulham, Social Services Area No. 2, Federal House, 1–2 Down Place, London, W6 9JH.

Brian Jarman MA DIC PhD FRCP FRCGP
Acheson Professor of General Practice
Department of General Practice, St Mary's Hospital Medical School, Lisson Grove Health Centre, Gateforth Street, London, NW8 8EG.

Matthijs Muijen MD MRCPsych
Research Worker and Honorary Senior Registrar
Institute of Psychiatry and Bethlem Royal and Maudsley Hospital, University of London, De Crespigny Park, London, SE5 8AF.

Fiona Ross BSc PhD RGN NDNCert
Lecturer
Department of Nursing Studies, King's College, University of London, 552 King's Road, London, SW10 0UA.

Alison While BSc MSc PhD SRN HVCert
Lecturer
Department of Nursing Studies, King's College, University of London, 552 King's Road, London, SW10 0UA.

Preface

The needs of inner city inhabitants are being increasingly acknowledged. Professionals working in inner cities are there to help individuals (children and adults) to maximize their opportunities and to cope with the difficulties in their lives. This book focuses on the needs of the inner city population, and outlines how professionals may facilitate in the course of their daily practice.

The book has followed a biographical approach with relevant experts contributing to the chapters. Chapter 1 sets the general scene with a brief overview of inner city problems. Chapter 2 examines the needs of pre-school children and provides ideas for supporting young families as they embark on parenthood. Chapter 3 discusses the needs of school children and offers examples of professional practice which meet these needs. Chapter 4 provides knowledge and information about young people (youth) and gives a brief account of facilities for young people. Chapter 5 discusses the nature of family life in inner cities and makes suggestions for improvement in individual professional practice. Chapter 6 reviews the difficulties of general practice provision and outlines the Government's most recent recommendations. Chapter 7 examines the evidence regarding increased mental health problems and describes an interesting project set up in conjunction with a well-known psychiatric hospital. Chapter 8 focuses on the needs of the elderly and how their needs and those of their carers may be met. Chapter 9 concludes the book and emphasizes that while there are many problems facing inner city community workers, there are also excellent examples of how practitioners have innovated to improve the service they are able to offer.

This book could not have been written without the commitment of the authors, for which I am most grateful. Thanks are also due to Heinemann Medical Books for encouraging this project and to Mary Fahy who always manages to make handwriting so legible. A special thank you to my husband,

Philip, for his constant encouragement and to my young sons, William and Edward, for leaving this manuscript in one piece!

A. E. W.
London, 1988

1

Introduction

ALISON WHILE

> Enough is known about the decay, poverty and socially unstable nature of inner city environments for us to suppose that they can exert strangely negative influences on many of the people who live in them.
>
> (Blakemore, 1983, p. 82)

This statement focuses attention upon the concern that currently pervades the public mind. Namely, the attributed association between inner city life and 'problems'. Indeed, during the last few years, urban problems have assumed an increasingly important place in the hierarchy of contemporary ills, with cities identified as exemplars of the dissolution of society. This concern has resulted in increasing Government intervention in urban economies, together with the realization by politicians of all parties to the potential and actual consequences of inner city neglect and decline.

THE BACKGROUND

Much of the housing of our inner cities is old and needs substantial repair and there is evidence that those living in inner cities have accommodation with poorer amenities and higher rates of overcrowding than elsewhere. One strategy for improving housing stock has been redevelopment, however, the time lag between moving people out for slum clearance and the availability of large sites for redevelopment has resulted in the destruction of existing communities and the dispersal of households. Further, much of the high-rise public housing built in the 1960s has left a legacy of social and structural problems for the

1980s. Indeed, some of these buildings have had to be demolished, while others have become notorious estates in which people fear to tread, with unenviable reputations and high vacancy rates.

The 1980 Housing Act introduced a new phenomenon to public sector housing; namely, the opportunity for council tenants to purchase their homes. However, it is relatively high income tenants who can afford to service mortgages and, further, highest rates of sales have been experienced in the better quality 'cottage' estates — it seems that less than 5% of sales have involved flats, although they constitute nearly a third of public sector housing stock. Indeed, the reduction in public sector expenditure has ignored the needs of the most vulnerable in the population, that is, the old, unemployed and one-parent families. Lawless and Brown (1986) have argued that current Government policies have exacerbated the inequalities in housing through the massive transfer in subsidies from the public to the owner-occupied sector.

However, much has changed in our inner cities since they were built, apart from the deterioration in housing provision. The size of inner city populations has declined dramatically since 1960 (Department of Environment, 1975) and employment opportunities, particularly in manufacturing, have fallen noticeably (Department of Employment, 1976). Interestingly, despite the overall prosperity of South-East England, London has suffered a greater decline in its manufacturing base as compared with other major conurbations. Further, inner cities are not attractive locations for entrepreneurs, who find that the high land costs and the unfavourable industrial structure and infrastructure can be avoided by development of their enterprises elsewhere. Employment statistics indicate that the main growth of employment involves the service sector which is predominantly female employment, much on a part-time basis. Indeed, this contributes to the evidence that approximately 40% of the unemployed live in the seven major metropolitan areas of the United Kingdom. The inner city populations also suffer from selective out-migration of younger and more skilled individuals, which leaves an increasingly ageing population dominated by individuals with limited industrial skills who are unable to command high wages.

Changes have occurred in the area of transport provision. The 1985 Transport Act introduced competitive tender to bus provision. While the Government believes this will improve services at the same time as reducing costs and subsidies, others have argued that it will increase the cost of local transport for the consumer together with increasing road congestion. Indeed, the problem of road congestion is particularly acute in London where traffic is frequently at a standstill. The evidence suggests, however, that car ownership has risen in cities, which has reduced the pressure for public transport, although the statistics indicate that most people in cities do not have access to a car. Therefore, buses serve an important function, especially for the 'car-less' inner city dweller; namely, the semi-skilled and unskilled, women, children and old people. Further, transport facilities have recently acquired a greater importance with changes in inner city retail provision. Inner-urban development programmes have tended to herald the loss of the cheap corner shop and its replacement by chain shores and superstores which are aimed at a higher income market and frequently located for the shopper who has the use of a car.

The particular difficulties in educational provision in inner cities is discussed in Chapter 3. However, like housing and employment, the educational needs of inner city inhabitants are less well provided for when comparisons are drawn with suburban education. Indeed, the high teacher turnover and the high proportion of children from very low income households is noteworthy, together with the increased concentration of learning and linguistic problems in inner city schools. Some have argued that the demise of inner city education is in part reflected in the high unemployment rates among young inner city dwellers who have failed to develop adequate skills for the labour market of the present. It has been accepted for many years that educational qualifications are closely related to occupation and income earned, so the issue of inner city education is an important one.

SOLUTIONS ?

Acknowledgement of the inner city problem caused the introduction of a number of urban experiments. It was argued that there were many advantages to the adoption of a more integrated approach to the management of urban areas. Lawless (1981) charts the development and execution of such policies; however, he wondered whether the sheer mechanics of preparing an agreed urban programme became more important on occasions than any results that might have been achieved!

This book does not attempt to offer macro solutions to the problems facing the inner cities, rather the authors have all addressed the issue of health needs for different groups of inner city residents. Each author has outlined examples of 'good practice' which might serve as a catalyst for the development of initiatives by professionals working in inner cities. It is hoped that the ideas put forward will be helpful to professionals as they pursue excellence in their work practice.

REFERENCES

Blakemore K. (1983). Ageing in the inner city: a comparison of old Blacks and Whites, in Jerrome D. (ed.), *Ageing in Modern Society*. London: Croom Helm.

Department of Employment (1976). *Employment in Metropolitan Areas.* **Unit for Manpower Studies**. London: Her Majesty's Stationery Office.

Department of Environment (1975). *Study of the Inner Areas of Conurbations*. London: Department of Environment.

Lawless P. (1981). *Britain's Inner Cities: Problems and Policies*. London: Harper and Row.

Lawless P. and Brown F. (1986). *Urban Growth and Change in Britain*. London: Harper and Row.

2

Early Childhood

ALISON WHILE

We consider '. . . that the disadvantages of birth and early
life cast long shadows forward'.

(DHSS, 1976, p. 3)

INTRODUCTION

Early childhood experiences are known to have a profound effect
upon future life. This chapter will explore the nature of these
experiences for children resident in inner cities and will also
review the health status of these children. However, an important section will explore how the health and social needs of inner
city children may be met by support provisions and provide
examples of innovations and initiatives in this field.

THE SITUATION OF FAMILIES WITH YOUNG
CHILDREN

A number of authors have argued that the decay, poverty and
socially unstable nature of inner city environments exert a
negative influence upon the inhabitants. Indeed, Madge (1982) in
a review has catalogued the range of physical, material, behavioural and social adversities inherent in growing up in an inner
city. Multiple and pervasive deprivation will clearly have its
effect upon children growing up in an inner city; indeed, it is an
especially important consideration regarding children in their
pre-school years who are most affected by their home environment because of their dependence upon the family for physical
care, emotional security and intellectual stimulation.

While the number of homes offering basic amenities has improved since the 1950s, the demise of the 'have-nots' has been exacerbated by the increasing affluence of other members of society so that relatively they have to endure poorer environments. The lack of adequate housing conditions has implications. All children require space – it is a necessity for the development of healthy family relationships and for expression through play and, further, poor housing conditions may not only cause poor health but also inhibit optimum care during episodes of childhood illness. Madge (1982) referred to the development of a social handicap among children from deprived families which she argued may endure throughout life – a point which has been raised by professionals working in inner city areas many times.

The housing market consists of two main sectors; the private (with either owner-occupation or rented occupation) and the public in which local authority tenancies fall. Different types of housing tenure are associated with unequal advantages and disadvantages. However, for the purposes of this chapter it is worth noting that private tenants are more likely than council tenants or owner-occupiers to live in poor housing conditions and also that a higher proportion of private tenants live in unfit dwellings. A recent survey undertaken by the author in Inner London found that most (48.7%) families with a child under two years of age lived in council accommodation with Housing Trusts (17.9%) providing another important source of accommodation. Owner-occupiers amounted to 16.8% of the families with a further 16.5% of families dependent upon the private rental market.

One of the changes in housing provision in the inner cities since World War II has been the removal of familiar but decaying terraced houses and their replacement by anonymous high-rise blocks of flats. The survey data confirmed this with flats being the most usual type of accommodation for young families (80.7%), houses being occupied by only 14.8% of the families. Approximately 5% of families were resident in bedsitter accommodation. The data also revealed that 16% of families had the use of only one bedroom. More detailed data of household conditions demonstrated that not all families had the use of reasonable cooking facilities – 6.9% of the sample either shared their kitchen or were dependent upon bedsitter cooking facilities. And while the vast majority of families had their own bathrooms, 6.7% of families had shared bathing facilities or no access to such facilities. The above statistics are reported in order to highlight the demise of some young families in our inner cities and to show that it cannot be assumed that material deprivation is a phenomenon of the past. Indeed, current and future changes in the management of public housing may result in the deterioration of standards in the public sector, although the Government has expressed a commitment in the maintenance of housing standards.

A common feature of young families in inner cities is the dependence of a sizeable minority upon emergency accommodation provided by local authorities under the 1985 Housing Act (Part III). Surveys have found 8–10% of families with young children requiring the services of Homeless Families Units. The length of time families spend in this type of accommodation is very variable; however, the available statistics suggest that stays are generally less than four months, although there is evidence that some families remain in bed and breakfast accommodation in excess of two years. Not only is this type of accommodation notoriously poor, but it is generally some distance from the community from which the families have come and is also not located in the community in which they will be permanently housed. Thus the families are socially isolated as well as materially deprived in terms of housing amenities which imposes great demands upon their personal resources as well as those of the neighbourhood in which they are transiently located. The particular needs of young families in this situation have been well reviewed by Rogers (1987) and in *Roof* (1987).

Inner city families are also renowned for their mobility as they seek to establish themselves in both the housing and employment markets. Mobility can be considered in two ways – number of home moves and movement between boroughs and district health authorities. The majority of families do not move their residences; however, in excess of 30% of families in certain inner cities move at least once when they have an infant under one year of age, and about 25% of families move at least once with older pre-school children. These statistics disguise evidence that there are different rates of moving home in different localities and the different rates of mobility of different groups of the population – immigrants are noted for their mobility. Interestingly, the majority of moves are a relatively short distance, giving rise to the national statistic that six out of ten moves are within $2\frac{1}{2}$ miles and approximately one in fifteen moves are greater than 50 miles. Inner city residents are more mobile than other residents, however, most moves do not involve a change in district health authority so that approximately only 16% of young families experience two district health authorities and only 4% of young families have lived in three or more district health authority areas.

The importance of acknowledging this mobility lies in the disruption it may cause to health promotion and surveillance activity. Changing of doctors, child health clinics, social service area and professional worker mean that professionals must be particularly conscientious about forwarding necessary information so that programmes of treatment and prevention may be continued. The use of a parent-held child health record and computerization of relevant information are two ways in which the problem of poor information transfer may be overcome. A further compounding factor in inner cities is the mobility of professional care workers themselves. The author found in her research that approximately half inner city families with children under two years of age had 3–5 different health visitors make home visits in a period of twenty-four months. One can therefore easily understand why families claim that they receive different and sometimes conflicting child-care advice, because this finding conceals whether or not the families saw the same or different health visitors when they attended child health clinic sessions.

However, poor housing together with high mobility are but two of the adverse social circumstances in inner cities which families with young children experience. Indeed, it is acknowledged that a number of factors associated with social disadvantage cluster together in inner cities and exert a negative effect upon family well-being. These factors include: maternal youthfulness, single parenthood, poverty, unemployment, Social Class V, cultural diversity and illiteracy in English. The importance of young maternal age lies in the reduced resources that younger people as parents have to offer their children and, further, reflects in general a lack of preparation for the role. Average maternal age on the birth of children is lower in inner cities than in suburbs and approximately 15% are below 20 years of age and some are still officially school children themselves. The particular difficulties of this group are addressed in the next chapter. Associated with young maternal age is single parenthood, and in a recent survey in the Inner London area 30% of young families were headed by a single parent. Thus, families with a single young mother may be very vulnerable as they strive to survive in a society in which the extended family offers very limited, if any, support.

Associated with single parenthood and unemployment is the experience of poverty. How much money a family has determines their access to goods and services and in so doing shapes their standard of living and influences their social status. Poverty has been shown to be associated with poor physical development in children and with many other indices of disadvantage, for example, inadequate housing, low educational attainment, problems in parenting and crime. Interestingly, the author's recent survey in the Inner London area found that 30% of young families had relied upon Supplementary Benefit payments as a source of family income; a further 6% of families had relied upon Unemployment or Sickness Benefit. The Black Report's compilation of research evidence (DHSS, 1980) conclusively demonstrated that poverty was a major determinant of health – further research regarding the North of England (Whitehead, 1987) and in Bristol (Townsend et al, 1984) confirm the association between limited family income (poverty) and poor health experience.

A group of families who require particular support are those whose breadwinner has been convicted of a crime and sent to prison. These families are deprived not only of a steady source of income derived from an employed parent, but also of the normal social relationships of family life. It has been argued by some that the children are innocent victims of the penal system. The lack of a named agency to deal with the problems of these children means that health professionals and others working in the community must offer whatever support they can. Roger Shaw's (1987) book is most useful and thought provoking.

Membership of an ethnic minority has few advantages in British society. Despite the efforts of the Commission for Racial Equality and legislative changes, all the evidence suggests that 'black' people do not experience the same opportunities as 'white' people. The importance of raising this point lies in the fact that most 'black' people live in our inner city areas and frequently come into contact with welfare professionals who might be able to offer guidance and support.

The clustering of adverse socio-economic factors must be considered as contributing to the inferior health experience of ethnic minorities. Townsend's (1979) survey found that 43% of households with a non-white member were in Social Classes IV and V as compared with 26% of the whole sample. Further, 14% of households with a non-white member were either in or on the margins of poverty compared to 9% of the whole sample, and 42% were defined as 'deprived' by the index used as compared with 16% of the whole sample. This finding complements the evidence that black workers are more vulnerable to unemployment than the white population, the consequences of which are increasingly acknowledged in terms of mental health morbidity.

An area in which immigrant families experience inferior opportunity is housing. Smith (1976) found that Asian households were more cramped than the indigenous population, a situation which continues to prevail because of three factors: (1) multi-occupation permits a number of earners to contribute to the high cost of private rental agreements; (2) the desire for large family units to remain together in a close-knit life style; (3) the limited consumer power of black people in the private rental market. Indeed, a report by the Commission for Racial Equality (1984) found evidence that black people were allocated poorer quality council housing than white people, despite claims by the borough to the contrary.

The inequalities of income, employment, housing and education opportunities experienced by ethnic minorities were considered by the House of Commons Home Affairs Committee (1981) and the evidence received by that Committee is an excellent source of reference. Further, the inferior social and home circumstances of children of immigrants has been documented by the National Child Development Study (Fogelman, 1983).

FAMILY STRESS

Under certain stressful conditions family members may behave in a positively harmful way to each other – the result is family violence. Recent publicity surrounding the death of Jasmine Beckworth in Brent has highlighted one of the unfortunate circumstances of families under stress and the need for health and community workers to be ever vigilant.

It is not my intention to develop this section on family stress and child abuse in any great detail. There are many excellent texts available to the reader, an example of which is Moore

(1985). Suffice to say that family stress can arise as a result of circumstances and factors relating to either the adults or the child. Stressors among parents include their immaturity, marital or relationship difficulties, single parenthood, unemployment and economic difficulties, and lack of knowledge about child-rearing. It must also be acknowledged that some children are more difficult than others to rear, for example, infants that are difficult to settle and/or feed and hyperactive children.

An interesting American study (Jason, 1983) has explored all 'murders' of children under 18 years of age. The deaths fell into two broad categories: (1) until about 3 years of age the deaths were predominantly of intra-familial origin and associated with bodily force and poorly defined precipitating events; (2) after 12 years of age the deaths were predominantly of extra-familial origin, involving weapons such as knives used during arguments or criminal acts, and probably represent children unsupervised in an adult environment; (3) between 3 and 12 years of age a mixture of these two types occurred. Indeed, before 12 years of age it seems that murders are perpetrated by those known to the child – parents, step-parents, other relatives and acquaintances, while after 12 years of age strangers and unidentified persons become important, although most important were acquaintances.

INFANT AND PRE-SCHOOL CHILD HEALTH

Vulnerable newborn infants

Even before an infant is born the importance of family back-ground comes into play. Indeed, it is an established fact that families of babies in Special Care Baby Units have more social problems than do those of normally sized babies. Further, the evidence of the British Births Survey (Chamberlain *et al*, 1975) suggested that babies born into Social Classes IV and V have a shorter gestation than those in the middle classes, with the difference being greater among unsupported mothers.

Evidence has also suggested that ethnic group is one of the most important factors influencing low birth-weight. The impor-tance of low birth-weight lies in its association with increased mortality and morbidity rates. Studies in the United States have found that nearly one in eight babies born to black mothers weigh 2500 grams or less. This is approximately twice as many as those born to white mothers, even when low family income and poor parental educational attainment are allowed for.

However, many studies of birth-weight around the world have found that babies born in developing countries weigh less than babies born elsewhere. The difference is particularly marked when babies from the Indian subcontinent are considered. Interestingly, babies from the Indian subcontinent are considerably lighter than European babies at term, although there is very little difference between the two groups before thirty-two weeks' gestation. It has been suggested that such babies are small-for-dates because of some factor constraining growth towards the end of pregnancy. A study in London found that Indian babies weighed, on average, 250 grams less than white babies, while the average weight of West Indian babies fell between that for white and Indian babies. It seems, therefore, that genetics plus short stature and poor nutrition have their part to play. Clearly, health professionals can do little to influence the former; however, they can do much to improve the latter and indeed the House of Commons Social Service Committee Report (1980) advocated concerted action to improve health care delivery (health surveillance and health promotion) to vulnerable groups. Recent years have seen the development of excellent campaigns to involve minority groups in health care. Examples of these are: the ten pilot schemes of the Asian Mother and Baby Campaign which will be reported by Vena Bahl of the DHSS and support groups for Asian women. These have been very successful in not only providing health promotion information but also improving the poor antenatal booking rate of this group.

INFANTS DURING THEIR FIRST YEAR OF LIFE

Central to consideration of infant mortality rates has been the evidence that, despite the steady improvement of infant mortality rates over the years, the social class gradient in health experience is more marked in Britain than in some comparable countries. The Black Report (DHSS, 1980) drew attention to these differentials which appeared uninfluenced by more than thirty years of a national health service expressly committed to offering equal care to all. Epidemiological evidence also demonstrates increased infant and child mortality rates in inner cities (for example, Glasgow and Edinburgh (Carstairs, 1981); Bristol

(Townsend *et al*, 1984)). Perhaps the most distresssing evidence was presented in a study of infant deaths in Inner London by Palmer *et al* (1980) which found that 37% of the deaths were attributed to diseases that are treatable. Indeed, it is known that post-neonatal mortality is influenced by 'social' as opposed to 'medical' factors.

However, not only are infant mortality rates higher in inner cities, but also infant morbidity rates are significantly higher. The author's research found a noticeably greater hospital contact rate among infants resident in an inner city district of London as compared with suburb residents. Associated with these findings was evidence that uptake of prophylactic care among infants requiring hospital care was markedly lower. Indeed, such infants were less likely to have attended child health clinics for assessments or immunizations and further were more likely to have been bottle-fed rather than breast-fed. While it is difficult to understand all the reasons for the poorer health of some infants, it was clear that some families were not benefiting in full from health service provision. It is particularly interesting that such families were frequently receiving social work support as well as normal health visiting support − it may have been that such families have many difficulties in their lives and therefore find themselves obliged to manage a series of crises so that prophylactic care is neglected while acute illness associated with hospitalization has to be managed.

PRE-SCHOOL CHILDREN

The prime causes of death in the first year of life, such as congenital abnormalities, are less important to childhood mortality, two-thirds of deaths being attributed to cancers, respiratory diseases and accidents. The social class differences are not particularly marked for cancers, however, proximity to installations handling nuclear material has been demonstrated as important by some recent research. While the proportion of childhood deaths from infective and respiratory diseases has fallen dramatically over time, a social class trend has remained, with children from the lower social classes having a significantly higher mortality rate.

However, accidents are the commonest cause of death after the first year of life and are responsible for 22% of all deaths between the ages of 1 and 4 years, rising to 40% of deaths of 5−

9-year-olds and older children. Causes of these accidental deaths vary according to the age of children; of particular significance are poisoning, burns and drowning among children under 5 years of age, while motor vehicle traffic accidents account for the majority of all accidental deaths in older children (OPCS, 1985). Social class trends have persisted over time regarding childhood accident rates and it is acknowledged that inner city residence in poor accommodation with its limited space for safe play mitigates against improvements in the depressing statistics. Evidence suggests that there is a need for continued efforts to educate parents about child safety and to persuade architects and planners to make provisions for safe areas for play.

While mortality rates are relatively low among pre-school children, childhood illness is an everyday experience of most families. Indeed, children are heavy users of general practitioner services, with family doctors seeing 98% of their under-five-year-old practice population within one year (R. C. G. P *et al*, 1986). Much evidence exists demonstrating a social class differential in childhood morbidity rates with lower social class children experiencing both more frequent and more severe illness episodes. Further confirmation of this inequality of experience can be found through an examination of hospital contact data where lower social group children are over-represented regarding hospital admission rates, outpatient appointments and attendance at Accident and Emergency Departments. The author's research also found greater hospital contact rates among inner city families as compared with suburban families, regardless of social class background. This in part may be a reflection of increased use of Accident and Emergency Departments for primary health care and less good general practitioner services in the inner city.

Prophylactic care is provided for children under 5 years of age through the health visiting and child health clinic service. However, recent data have confirmed the Court Report findings (DHSS, 1976) that children over 1 year of age are infrequent attenders of child health clinics and rarely see health visitors except perhaps on an annual basis. This is particularly true of children in inner city areas where health visitors have many urgent demands upon their time which force routine health surveillance into the background. It is therefore not surprising that a significant number of children are entering school with treatable problems which have apparently not received attention.

Indeed, a survey carried out in 1983 (MacFarlane and Pillay, 1984) revealed an immense variation in service provision which was not reflective of any criteria such as proportion of ethnic minority population, rates of unemployment or other demographic characteristics. However, it is recognized that services can be more effective if specific local situations and needs are acknowledged. For example, an inquiry into infant deaths in Sheffield has led to a more flexible health visiting provision and improved communication of information between all those, including parents, concerned with a child's health (Jepson et al, 1983). Substantial changes have also been introduced in a child health clinic in Nottingham, with the result that an older and more deprived pre-school child population used the clinic services and more treatable medical problems were detected (Nicoll et al, 1986).

Also of interest is the evidence from the research of Bax and his colleagues (1980) in an Inner London district, which indicated a relationship between adverse social circumstance and particularly maternal stress and health and behaviour of the pre-school child. They further found that an excess of respiratory infections, developmental delay and behavioural problems were interrelated. Clearly, there is a need for sensitive service provision if the needs of inner city children are to be met.

SUPPORT FOR FAMILIES

The needs of families in our inner cities have been briefly outlined. In this section the author will attempt to provide examples and ideas of how some of these needs (health and social) can be met by professionals working in the community.

There are now various examples of ways in which health visitors, despite resource shortages, are responding to local community needs. These include workshops for parents, out-of-hours services for crying babies, evening clinics and 24-hour health visiting services and positive discrimination in health visiting for disadvantaged families. Indeed, such health visitor work is being evaluated as part of the Bristol Child Development Project (Barker, 1981).

Good communication is important to any service, however, it is particularly important to the child health services if a good standard of provision is to be maintained. The adoption of parent-held child health records may in part overcome the difficulties of information transfer – this does not merely mean the issue of such records, but their active use by professionals offering care and advice to families. It is clear, therefore, that professionals themselves must be conscientious and keep colleagues informed of when they suspect family difficulties if the recent tragedies in Brent and Greenwich are to be avoided in the future. Good teamwork founded upon sound communication is an asset to inner city health provision.

The work of social service departments is invaluable in inner cities, however, so great are the demands made upon them that only the 'lucky' families receive social work casework. In the author's survey in Inner London, in excess of 25% of families have experienced the support of a social worker during the first two years of the child's life. Interestingly, some of the social worker support was given by voluntary agencies such as Family Service Unit, Welcare, RNIB, and some families continued to make contact with hospital social workers. A small number of families gained support on a regular basis from the probation service, education welfare officers and a Sister of Charity who has devoted her later life to the particular needs of immigrants from North Africa, especially Moroccans. The contribution of NSPCC social workers can also be most helpful in supporting families through difficult times.

The financial plight of some inner city families has already been discussed. However, these difficulties are in part reflective of the shortage of child care provision. For many years it has been recognized that local authority day nursery provision is inadequate to meet the large need among inner city parents. Indeed, so great is the demand for places that a priority system operates by which only potential abusing families or families with significant difficulties gain places in this scarce resource. This situation has two consequences: namely, the day nursery child population is composed almost exclusively of children with difficulties, some of which are the consequence of family problems; and more importantly, families with 'normal' children who require day care for their pre-school children are forced to make less than satisfactory arrangements with childminders. Evidence in the 1970s suggested that as many as a third of mothers of children under 5 years were unable to find the help they felt they needed outside the home in raising their children.

The background to this demand in the inner cities has been the increasing number of work opportunities for women, financial pressures, an increase in the number of single parent families, the disintegration of the extended family as a means of support for the nuclear family, the new status of women, together with the stress and isolation of urban living. Indeed, depression has been shown to be fairly widespread among young mothers at home. However, despite the need for child care, remarkably few children gain day nursery places – nationally, about 1% of the under-five population as compared with approximately 13% of the inner city pre-school child population. A similar number of children are *known* to be looked after by childminders – about 4% nationally as compared with about 12% in the inner city. While a well planned experience stretches the under-fives and gives them confidence for their school life, a poor experience can have a lasting detrimental effect. In view of this, the findings of Mayall and Petrie (1983) are disheartening; namely, only a third of children in their survey were looked after by minders whose premises and equipment were up to official standards. Indeed, they found that the use of a childminder was a chancy business, with much variation in standards regarding environment, including equipment and the quality of child care. Further, childminding arrangements also tended to be unstable, with children frequently moving from one minder to another. And of particular relevance to the inner cities was their finding that mothers in manual work and from abroad tended to get a poorer deal, with ethnic minority families making much greater use of unregistered minders whose credentials are known to be questionable.

A source of support for some families lies in their membership of groups. There is some evidence that support groups can be of great help. There are a variety of contexts in which they arise: namely, a support group for families sharing a particular situation, for example, a child with a handicap (Contact-A-Family or MENCAP); a support group under the auspices of a particular organization (National Childbirth Trust, Gingerbread); a support group developed by care professionals, examples of which include postnatal support groups initiated by health visitors and their colleagues, and support groups initiated by child guidance clinics and social work provision, including the NSPCC. It is thought that membership of such groups among families with pre-school children may be as great as 20% in the inner cities where the opportunity exists, however, approximately a further 6% of families have a fleeting membership of support groups but on finding their needs are not met or being unable to sustain a commitment, allow their membership to lapse. Perhaps inner city care workers could do more to facilitate the development of support groups.

Playgroups are another source of support and fulfil a variety of local needs. They can be helpful in combating the anonymity and isolation of high rise flats, together with 'mixing' in racially varied neighbourhoods. Further, they provide the opportunity for safe play for 3–5 year old children and offer a wider range of play materials than any single family could sustain. The social benefits to children and parents are acknowledged, with children having the opportunity to extend their social contact beyond their kinship group in preparation for school life and parents supporting one another through their commitment to the play-group. The number of playgroups in any neighbourhood varies over time since their inauguration and continued existence depends upon the commitment of a number of individuals, usually mothers. However, it is thought that approximately 18% of children under 5 years of age attend playgroups. And it appears that some children gain experience outside the home through their attendance at nursery schools (7%) and reception classes of primary schools (8%). The extent of this provision depends upon local education authority funding and support and is known to vary considerably nationwide.

The contribution of care workers in the inner cities is variable. The particular difficulties of providing a good general practitioner service is discussed in a later chapter, however, the under-five population is very vulnerable to episodes of illness as they develop their immune systems and investigate their environments which are full of potential hazards so that accidents are a frequent occurrence. It is thought, however, that approximately 20% of inner city families do not have a general practitioner upon whom they can call, with immigrant families having a lower registration rate than the indigenous population. The particular problems of homeless families and their more frequent mobility have resulted in perhaps an even poorer service being provided for this needy group. The chapter by Brian Jarman (pp. 94–115) will be useful to the reader in a consideration of the problems of the general practitioner service. The contribution of health visitors is also variable, although some examples of practice developments have been mentioned earlier in this section. One difficulty, however, remains that of resource shortage, with a dependence upon more recently qualified staff — perhaps health visiting in inner cities would become more attractive if health visitors were permitted to develop different ways of working in response to local needs. For example, given time in which to develop their own practice through fostering a support group or an out-of-hours service for crying babies. Similarly, resource problems plague social service departments and perhaps they too could examine the workloads of their caseworkers so that they too are able to develop a less transient team of social workers who will be more familiar with the neighbourhood, both its needs and its resources.

CONCLUSION

The needs of young inner city families are many, however, while accepting that resources are likely to be limited in the foreseeable future, it is hoped this chapter has provided some ideas how care worker practice could respond to these needs and innovate support provisions to improve family and child well-being.

REFERENCES

Barker W. (1981). Child Development. Second Progress Report. Bristol: University of Bristol.

Bax M., Hart H. and Jenkins S. (1980). *The Health Needs of the Preschool Child*, Thomas Coram Research Unit. London: Institute of Education, University of London.

Carstairs V. (1981). Multiple deprivation and health state. *Community Medicine*, **3** (1), 4–13.

Chamberlain R., Chamberlain G., Howlett B. and Claireaux A. (1975). *British Births 1970*. Volume I: The First Week of Life. London: Heinemann Medical.

Department of Health and Social Security (1976). *Fit for the Future*. Report of the Committee on Child Health Services. Cmnd 6684 (Chairman: Professor S. D. M. Court). London: Her Majesty's Stationery Office.

Department of Health and Social Security (1980). *Inequality in Health*. Report of a research working group (Chairman: Sir Douglas Black). London: Department of Health and Social Security.

Ghodsian M. and Essen J. (1983). Children of immigrants: social and home circumstances. Part of Chapter 3: Immigrants, in Fogelman K. (ed.), *Growing Up in Great Britain*. London: Macmillan.

House of Commons (1980). Second Report from the Social Services
    Committee. Session 1979/80. *Perinatal and Neonatal Mortality*.
    Volume I: Report (Chairman: Mrs R. Short). London: Her Majesty's
    Stationery Office.
House of Commons (1981). *Report of Home Affairs Committee on Racial
    Disadvantage*. Volume I: Fifth Report (Chairman: Sir G. Page).
    London: Her Majesty's Stationery Office.
Jason J. (1985). Child homicide spectrum. *American Journal of Diseases in
    Childhood*, **137** (6), 578–81.
Jepson M. E., Taylor E. M. and Emery J. L. (1983). Identification of
    failures in the child health services by means of confidential
    enquiries into infant deaths. *Maternal and Child Health*, **8**, (1), 26–31.
MacFarlane J. A. and Pillay U. (1984). Who does what, and how much
    in the pre-school child health services in English. *British Medical
    Journal*, **289**, 851–2.
Madge N. J. H. (1982). Growing up in the inner city. *Journal of the Royal
    Society of Health*. **102** (6), 261–5.
Mayall B. and Petrie P. (1983). *Childminding and Day Nurseries*. London:
    Heinemann Educational.
Moore J. G. (1985). *The ABC of Child Abuse Work*. London: Gower.
Nicoll A. *et al* (1986). The child health clinic: results of a new strategy
    of community care in a deprived area. *Lancet* **1**, (8481), 15th March.
    606–8.
OPCS (1985). *Mortality Statistics 1984*. London: Her Majesty's Statio-
    nery Office.
Palmer S. R., Wiggins R. D. and Bewley B. R. (1980). Infant deaths in
    Inner London: a health care planning team study. *Community
    Medicine*, **2**, 102–8.
Rogers R. (1987). No place like home. *Childright*. June 11–14.
Roof (1987). July/August issue.
Royal College of General Practitioners, OPCS and DHSS (1986).
    Morbidity Statistics for General Practice 1981–1982. Third National
    Study. London: Her Majesty's Stationery Office.
Shaw R. (1987). *Children of Imprisoned Fathers*. London: Hodder &
    Stoughton.
Smith D. (1976). *Facts of Racial Disadvantage: a national survey*. London:
    Political and Economic Planning Report.
Townsend P. (1979). *Poverty in the United Kingdom*. Harmondsworth:
    Allen Lane and Penguin.
Townsend P., Simpson D. and Tibbs N. (1984) *Inequalities of Health in
    the City of Bristol*. Bristol: University of Bristol.
Whitehead M. (1987). *The Health Divide: Inequalities in Health in the
    1980's*. London: Health Education Council.

3

School Children

ALISON WHILE

Children who grow up in poverty or squalor, whose homes are grossly overcrowded, or who live in decaying inner-city neighbourhoods ... such children are in different ways 'disadvantaged'.

(para. 1.44, DHSS, 1976)

INTRODUCTION

The school years are an important period in all individuals' lives. An attempt will be made to address pertinent issues during this period of the life span. The chapter will examine school provision, health needs and support provision. The research evidence, however, suggests that educational provision in inner cities faces many difficulties and that a disproportionate number of disadvantaged and maladjusted children attend inner city schools. Further, improved medical management has resulted in changes in health needs among school children, although accidents remain an important cause of both mortality and morbidity. And increasingly, the adoption of unhealthy behaviours by school children poses important challenges for professional workers and changes in practice will be needed. The last section of this chapter outlines potential support for school children and their families.

SCHOOL LIFE

The pupil population of inner London contains a large number of disadvantaged children. In addition, about 40%

are from ethnic minority groups and one in ten of all pupils
speak a mother tongue which is not English. Significant parts
of the area suffer from urban decay and some have changing
populations.

(DES, 1980)

While this statement refers to the situation in London, similar
educational needs are to be found in other inner cities, although
the statistical evidence suggests that the magnitude of the
problem is peculiar to London.

It has been suggested that disadvantaged children and (sometimes) schools are placed together. However, much attention is
focused upon educational achievements as represented in external examination passes rather than the whole range of educational achievements which are less measurable and more subtle.
It is interesting that inspectors' reports of many inner London
schools often acknowledge the strength of the schools in
stimulating creativity, initiative, cooperation and social concern
among pupils – qualities which are not easily assessed through
the formal education system. However, the fact remains that
much survey evidence has found poor scholastic attainment, high
absenteeism and fewer numbers of children remaining in education beyond the minimum school-leaving age.

The importance of considering schooling lies in the fact that
the level of attainment reached by a child on leaving school
usually has a profound influence on his or her future life chances;
that is, choice of employment and style of living. While clearly
this chapter is not the place to examine inner city schooling in
depth, some acknowledgement of the issues and problems is
pertinent. One of the areas of concern in inner city schools is the
behavioural standards exhibited by pupils – a concern which
gives the impression that it is more difficult of teach and learn in
the inner city compared with the outer city counterpart.

Underlying this phenomenon appears to be a higher prevalence of maladjustment in inner city schools. For example, Rutter
(1976) found that the incidence of maladjustment was twice as
high in inner London as compared with its incidence in the Isle of
Wight. Further, this research also found that the reading scores
of maladjusted pupils were far inferior to pupils classified as
normal. Indeed, the evidence suggests that inner city schools
have both more disadvantaged children and more maladjusted
children than other schools and as a consequence inevitably more

children appear to have poor levels of attainment. Clearly, the particular educational and social needs of inner city children need to be addressed.

The problems of educational provision are further compounded by three issues relating to teachers, namely: the difficulty in recruiting teachers in inner city schools; the difficulty in retaining teachers in inner city schools; and the difficulty in recruiting and retaining experienced teachers. The issue of teacher recruitment is a critical one and the consequence of high turnover rates for individual schools should not be underestimated – the combination of a high staff turnover coupled with a few teachers with more than a limited amount of teaching experience is far from ideal in inner city areas where demands upon teachers' skills are so great. Indeed, the stress of the situation probably causes further teacher turnover as individual teachers seek to find a more stable environment in which to exercise their skills. And further many would argue that the recent industrial unrest in schools has not been helpful in boosting morale and may have further exacerbated the situation.

Numerous studies have examined the relationship between school characteristics and average levels of attainment. Of particular note is the difference between reading attainment and rates of teacher turnover – high rates of turnover being associated with inferior reading attainment (Rutter, 1976). However, it appears that material features of schools such as location, state of repair, age of buildings, resources per pupil head, are of negligible importance (Rutter and Madge, 1976), while the social climate may be more influential. Pupils have been found to make better progress in schools rated by both teachers and pupils as placing a high value on achievement. Rutter *et al* (1975) have argued that the social structure and the stability of the school are important. Others have argued that the skills and experience of teachers, the quality of teacher-pupil relationships, the use of incentives and the responsibility given to pupils are also important (Rutter and Madge, 1976). Interestingly, Richardson *et al* (1983) reported that significantly higher attainments were found where schools showed concern for regular parent-teacher meetings, although the National Child Development Study limited its measurement of attainment to the performance in two standard tests, one in reading and the other in mathematics, and further sought to describe the status quo rather than what can be done to improve educational attainment.

Some of the findings of the National Child Development Study (Essen and Wedge, 1982) are worth consideration in the context of the inner city school. Of particular concern was the large proportion of disadvantaged 16-year-olds who were assessed by their teachers as being unable to do everyday calculations necessary for shopping and as being unable to read well enough to cope with everyday needs. The study found that disadvantaged children were ten times more frequently lacking these basic skills as compared with ordinary children. Indeed, the continued influence of 'disadvantage' was confirmed by this longitudinal research: namely, children who are ever in adverse circumstances (single parenthood, poor housing, etc.) tend to have relatively poor educational attainment at 16 years, even if their conditions have improved by that age. The research suggests that the difference in attainment between disadvantaged and ordinary children accumulate during adolescence, with differences that existed at 11 years increasing during the secondary school period.

While most children are educated in normal schools, some children experience particular difficulties in the educational system. Wedge and Essen (1982) in their report of the National Child Development Study data found that 1 in 20 of disadvantaged 11-year-olds were said to be educationally subnormal as compared with 1 in 150 of ordinary children. The follow-up data at 16 years of age revealed slightly greater contrasts, with 5.5% of all disadvantaged children being educated in ESN(M) schools which was nine times as many as the incidence among ordinary children (0.6%). The age of recognition of special educational needs was also related to whether the children were disadvantaged or not, with the long-term disadvantaged being particularly prejudiced in this respect (Essen and Wedge, 1982).

The difficulty of providing education for children from different cultures has recently caused public debate and concern, with the difficulties of racial integration in Manchester being the subject of a confidential report by John MacDonald, QC. The detailed exploration of these issues does not have a place in this chapter, however, some pertinent research findings will be briefly outlined from the National Child Development Study. The data revealed that second-generation immigrant children had better educational performance scores than first-generation immigrant children. The scholastic ability of second-generation Asians was particularly striking. West Indian children also had improved scores, although their scores remain considerably lower than any of the other immigrant groups. Essen and Ghodsian (1983) had two main conclusions, namely: immigrants' relatively poor attainment was a reflection of their social circumstances, and secondly, poorer school performance is generally only found among first-generation immigrants and is therefore relatively short-lived and language-specific. Indeed, their findings have considerable implications for the appropriate education for new immigrants so that their language needs and cultural adjustment needs are addressed through the provision of sensitive help.

The consumer view of education is easily overlooked, however, care workers can learn much about the needs of the community they serve through soliciting the 'client perspective'. Much anecdotal literature exists — an interesting consumer perspective may be read in Field's (1977) book. The four consumers clearly felt they had gained little from their school indeed, David's conclusions are salutory:

> I can't say I've got something out of school because I haven't got much. All the things I need I didn't get, like maths and English. I got woodwork but that's about all I got out of it, I didn't get nothing else. It's been a hard time for me.
>
> (p. 89, Field, 1977)

This brief review of the educational needs and provision has highlighted some of the shortcomings which currently prevail. It is unlikely that there will be a massive change in resources in the near future, however, this review has suggested relatively minor changes in practice could improve the situation. The concerns of teachers need addressing and perhaps workshops in the management of stress would improve attrition and turnover rates. The particular and continuing needs of long-term disadvantaged children also need addressing, with perhaps the school health service providing greater support. Indeed, the school nurse's role has much to offer the education service. She/he may be able to assist in the cultural adjustment of new immigrants through becoming a link person between the school and the home.

CHILDHOOD MORTALITY AND MORBIDITY

The incidence of infectious diseases has declined and further improved medical management has increased the survival rate of many sick children, so that more children are living with chronic disease, disabilities and handicaps. Data from the General Household Survey show increasing reports of long-standing illness in children and young people of both sexes (OPCS, 1986a).

However, there is evidence that some aspects of physical health have improved over the years. For example, children of both sexes were taller in 1981 as compared with 1972 (Rona and Chinn, 1984). But this improvement has occurred with an increased incidence of obesity (Stark et al, 1986). Further, it seems that anorexia nervosa may present a serious health problem to a small but increasing number of adolescent girls (about 1%). Indeed, this increase in the number of children with extremes of thinness and fatness suggests that new areas of physical health need active management, although the evidence suggests that successful management is difficult to attain.

Survey evidence has also found a dramatic improvement in dental health with a much reduced incidence of dental decay (Todd and Dodd, 1985). Interestingly, the decrease in dental decay has been most marked in younger children, although half the children currently entering school show signs of dental decay. However, the uptake of dental care is variable, with evidence from the National Child Development Study demonstrating a strong social gradient – disadvantaged children being less likely to have visited a dentist in the last year (65% of the long-term disadvantaged as compared with 88% of ordinary children) (Wedge and Essen, 1982). The incidence of dental care also reflects different dietary habits among school children, greater consumption of sugary products being associated with increased dental decay. Such dietary preferences are known to be exercised by disadvantaged children as an attempt at calorie filling; however, continued health promotion and education efforts have the potential to change these habits.

The experience of poor health is not only unpleasant, but may also affect the child's ability to function and to respond to learning opportunities. For example, absence from school through ill-health may result in healthier peers managing their school work with greater ease than their less fortunate classmate. Essen and Wedge (1983) found that at 11 years disadvantaged children missed more school for medical reasons than ordinary children, and similar findings pertained at 16 years of age. Interestingly, at 16 years of age the disadvantaged children suffered an increased incidence of bronchitis, which Essen and Wedge argued was related to either the longer period these children had spent in poor environmental conditions or to their acquired smoking habits. The development of unhealthy be- haviours will be discussed in greater depth later in this chapter.

Ethnic minority groups have special health problems, how- ever, the enumeration of these does not have a place in this chapter. Suffice to say that genetically determined disease may occur with sufficient frequency and severity to constitute an important health problem among some groups. For example, sickle-cell anaemia occurs in about 1:400 children in the Afro- Caribbean community. And where marriages are common between first or second cousins, recessively determined disorders occur with greater frequency than where such practices are rare. Among children from Asia, two nutritional disorders, iron- deficiency anaemia and rickets, are more common and may be diagnosed either in infancy or childhood. Tuberculosis is also more common among people from Asia, making the continued vaccination of this group of children important. And tropical diseases such as malaria, worm and intestinal infections are also more frequently experienced by Asian children who have lived in or visited the Indian subcontinent. This increased incidence of certain types of ill-health should be borne in mind by practi- tioners who work with these groups in inner cities.

Although infectious diseases have ceased to be such an important cause of ill-health in children, some infections continue to take their toll. Sexually transmitted diseases remain an important cause of morbidity in young people, however, their incidence is relatively rare under 16 years of age, but interest- ingly 34% of cases in females occurred under 20 years of age. The importance of rapid diagnosing and successful treatment of sexually transmitted diseases lies in the prevention of the long- term consequences, which include infertility, neurological prob- lems and chronic arthritis. The need for sensitive services to meet the needs of this part of the population are therefore crucial in the strategy to reduce the consequences of these diseases to a minimum − some health districts have developed excellent examples of practice and there is an argument for providing a screening service together with counselling at family planning clinics. School children in particular sometimes wonder where they may seek family planning advice without consultation with their parents; the difficulty in knowing where to go sometimes results in accidental pregnancies. The danger of rubella infection during early pregnancy has long been recognized and aggressive promotion of the uptake of the vaccination is an important contribution to the well-being of future babies. A small project (Smith and Fellner, 1985) has demonstrated that an active role by school nurses in the promotion of a rubella vaccination programme can greatly improve the uptake rates.

Accidents are an important cause of both morbidity and mortality. Motor vehicle accidents account for the majority of all accidental deaths among school children, with the mortality rate being particularly high among boys in the 15–19 year age group. However, the subsequent morbidity to accidents is probably more important as it not only causes absence from school, but also hospital admission and perhaps long-term disability. Hospital care is less disruptive in later years of childhood, nevertheless, for all children it is a dreaded experience and for many has few happy memories, with separation from normal home life and the endurance of intrusive procedures. The first report of the National Child Development Study (Davie *et al*, 1972) revealed that by 7 years of age about 10% of the study children had been admitted to hospital for a home accident and a further 10% had been admitted for accidental injuries other than those sustained at home or on the road. The follow-up report of the same children at 11 years revealed a social gradient, namely, the disadvantaged 11-year-olds were more likely than their ordinary contemporaries to have had an accident requiring hospital contact (admission or Accident and Emergency Department treatment) (Wedge and Essen, 1982). The difference in the frequency of accidents was accounted for by home accidents where burns and scalds took their toll. By 16 years of age the social gradient present among the accident rates at 11 years had almost disappeared, although the long-term disadvantaged were slightly more likely to have had an accident in the home and to have had more flesh wounds or burns than other children (Essen and Wedge, 1982). The change in the incidence of accidents is probably accounted for by increasing maturity resulting in hazards being avoided. However, the evidence suggests that further promotion of home safety and child awareness of potential hazards could improve the child accident statistics.

As certain causes of morbidity have decreased over the years, other conditions have assumed greater importance. The evidence about the incidence of child abuse is not conclusive (Addy, 1985), however, it seems that the most serious injuries have decreased, although there is a large number of injuries in total. This in part may be due to heightened awareness of the potential problem which has caused an increase in diagnosis of cases, particularly among children with less serious injuries. Sexual abuse of children is also increasingly recognized and it has been suggested that about 10% of women were sexually abused as children (Porter, 1984). The report of the Leeds Child Abuse Team's work makes interesting reading (Wild, 1986). They made a definite diagnosis of sexual abuse in 104 children in 1985; most cases had occurred in girls and the average age of the victims was 8.5 years. The promotion of self-empowerment among primary school children may improve these dismal statistics — both teachers and school nurses could develop programmes to this end, and perhaps voluntary children's groups such as those run under the auspices of the St John Ambulance Brigade, the Baden Powell movement and the Boys' and Girls' Brigade could also develop similar self-assertion programmes.

CHILDREN WITH TROUBLES

The adoption of unhealthy behaviours such as smoking, alcohol consumption and drug-taking are an acknowledged problem among some school children. The number of notifications of drug users and admissions to psychiatric care with drug-related problems have risen over the years (OPCS, 1986b). Although most notifications are in the 20–24-year age group, the numbers under 20 years are alarming. And further concern is warranted by the statistic that the vast majority of drug-users are dependent on heroin (alone or in combination), and that the figures only represent the minority of drug-users who are seeking treatment for their problem. Perhaps a more common problem among school children is solvent abuse — it is thought to occur most frequently among boys aged 13–15 years as a group activity (British Medical Journal, 1985). A scene-setting paper by McKerlie et al (1983) will be particularly useful to community workers not very familiar with the problem, and Cameron's (1985) description of a particular clinic may provide ideas of how a clinic can be managed. Further information for community workers may be sought from the Institute for the Study of Drug Dependence. However, accurate prevalence figures of solvent abuse are impossible to collect, with much variation between schools and in different years, although the level of abuse appears to rise in the summer months. Its importance lies, however, in the increasing death toll associated with the activity (Anderson et al, 1986).

More and more children are also known to drink alcohol and an increasing number of alcohol-related problems are being found in children (Plant et al, 1985). Further, alcohol plays an important role in road traffic accidents, and these accidents account for more than half of all male deaths among 15–19-year-olds (Havard, 1986). Moreover, health promotion work in this field will undoubtedly improve the sombre statistics.

Another unhealthy behaviour adopted by some school children is cigarette smoking. Dobbs and Marsh's (1985) survey revealed that 19% of school children between 11 and 16 years in England and Wales had smoked in 1982, 11% claimed they smoked regularly and 8% claimed they only smoked occasionally. They found little difference between the sexes, although the boys appear to experiment with cigarette smoking at an earlier age than the girls. Reid (1985) has reviewed strategies for reducing the prevalence of smoking among teenagers; he particularly recommends that educational programmes should begin at about 8–10 years of age, with high priority being given to the eduation of the 11–13-year age group. It seems that programmes based on education for personal growth are of more value than information packages. While Essen and Wedge (1982) found few health differences among the 16-year-old children in their study, they found that disadvantaged children were significantly more likely to smoke cigarettes as compared with ordinary children and in part they thought it may have explained the increased evidence of school absence due to bronchitis in this group.

A particularly difficult problem for some school children is bedwetting. The research is conclusive in finding a greater incidence of the problem among disadvantaged children (Davie et al, 1972; Essen and Wedge, 1982) and further it has been found to be associated with degree of social adjustment – poor adjustment being associated with greater incidence of bedwetting. Indeed, Wedge and Essen (1982) found that the disadvantaged children were three times more likely to bed-wet as compared with ordinary children. The management of this problem poses immense problems for both their families and the children themselves, indeed, the demanding home routine for maintaining hygiene standards inevitably delays departure to school so that it is hardly surprising that school attendance rates of sufferers are notoriously poor. Sensitive help for families is of paramount importance if they are to be assisted. A discussion paper, 'Eneuresis in School Children', produced by the Family Service Unit, is a most helpful contribution to the understanding of the problem and how it may be tackled.

Poor school attendance, however, may not be due to eneuresis and the stigmatizing and scapegoating which may go with it. It appears that occasional infrequent truancy is relatively common; Belsen (1975) found half his sample of boys had engaged in it at some time and in the National Child Development Study a similar proportion of children at 16 years had also engaged in truancy (Fogelman, 1976). However, severe and persistent truancy is less prevalent, with research evidence ranging from 8 to $\frac{1}{2}$% of school pupils, with an increased incidence among more senior secondary school pupils. Truancy has been found to be associated with age, sex, home environment, particular schools, poor educational attainment, delinquency and psychiatric disturbance (Berg, 1985). It is more prevalent among teenage boys and is more common in families in poor social circumstance, particularly poor housing (Tibbenham, 1983). Berg (1985) has outlined its management in some detail, however, lack of evaluative studies does not permit a suggestion as to the most effective management approach. Occasionally, school refusal may be confused with truancy. Hill's (1983a) article makes a most useful contribution to the understanding of the difference between the two problems, and in essence, school refusal is associated with other emotional symptoms, while truancy is classically associated with other antisocial behaviours. Like the management of truancy, the management of school refusal requires sound professional skill – the strategies which may be employed are described by Hill (1983b).

Although there is evidence of increased psychiatric morbidity among adult inner city residents, the incidence of severe mental illness among inner city children is difficult to assess. However, Rutter (1976) found a higher prevalence of maladjustment among Inner London pupils, and the National Child Develop-

ment Study found an increased incidence of poor social adjustment among disadvantaged children (Essen and Wedge, 1982).
With this background it is worth noting that the rates for suicide
among children and adolescents have increased, especially
among older boys (McClure, 1984). The possibility of severe
psychological problems among school children is therefore a
consideration for all those working with this age group.

This section is not intended to offer an exploration of the
exhaustive list of potential difficulties encountered in school life
and hence no attempt is made to address the issue of delinquency. Other texts, such as Hoghughi (1983), explore this
problem. However, with over 1200 girls under 16 years becoming mothers each year in England and Wales, schoolgirl motherhood is an important phenomenon. Its importance lies predominantly in the dismal statistics associated with it, namely, the high
rates of mortality of the resultant children, prematurity, low
birth-weight, stunted growth and developmental delay and non-
accidental injury (Black, 1986). There are far-reaching effects of
early motherhood, for example, cessation of education and loss
of status as a child for the mother. One study found that only a
quarter of teenage mothers actually planned to get pregnant and
half were upset to learn they were pregnant. Some have argued
that the increased pregnancy rate among under-16-year-olds has
been caused by the confusion surrounding the Gillick judgement,
so that some school children are reluctant to seek contraception
from the general practitioner because they are unsure whether he
will keep their confidence and not tell their parents. It seems that
once girls have had intercourse without any pregnancy resulting,
they can develop an unreal sense of immunity, indeed, the
availability of more information has not resulted in a greater use
of contraceptives because the raw experience of the teenage girls
does not relate to the dry facts of intercourse and the risk of
pregnancy. Another worrying aspect of teenage motherhood is
their poor participation in antenatal care, together with the
evidence that there is a high prevalence of smoking among this
group and that they are less likely to give up smoking during
their pregnancy. The particularly poor demise of their offspring
is also emphasized by the evidence of poverty (Williams *et al*,
1987). Black (1986) has argued that since most pregnant school-
girls live in large cities, it would be possible to develop special
provisions for them. An example of such a provision is Park
View House, a day school run by Sheffield Education Authority

as part of its hospital and home education service. This provision in Sheffield ensures that girls continue their education as well as acquiring mothering skills. The girls sit at least three CSEs so that they can enter the labour market with some evidence of educational success. Similar projects have been developed elsewhere. Two other examples of special provisions are the antenatal classes for teenagers only at King's College Hospital, London, and the Health and Counselling Group for pregnant teenagers in Hackney, London. Interestingly, a project in the United States found that return to education was more important in preventing further pregnancies than providing contraceptives.

SUPPORT FOR SCHOOL CHILDREN AND THEIR FAMILIES

A recent survey of London school children found that many are left to fend for themselves after school and during the school holidays while their parents are at work (Petrie and Logan, 1986). One in six 7-year-olds and one in three 11-year-olds are left alone, most being left for between three and four hours at a time. The survey mothers said they had little choice because local authorities offered so little out-of-school provision. A directory of out-of-school schemes for working parents in London is available through the National Out of School Alliance and although there is an immense variation in provision, all cities provide some support for working parents.

Since the 1944 Education Act there has been a statutory obligation for health authorities to make a health provision for school children. However, there are a number of problems with the school health service which were acknowledged in the Court Report (DHSS, 1976). Firstly, it has a purely advisory role with reliance upon curative branches of the National Health Service to provide treatment facilities, and, secondly, information transfer between general practitioners and the school health service is very poor. As a consequence, children and families frequently do not benefit from an integrated approach to health care provision with treatment being provided under the auspices of general practitioner care and with limited, if any, input from experts in educational medicine. The urgent need for improved liaison between schools and the home makes a strong case for child–parent held records. While school doctors make an important contribution to the school health service, the reality is that school nurses are the constant figures representing health provision in schools. Health interviews carried out by school nurses appear not only to be effective in surveillance work, but are also preferred by children, while providing an excellent opportunity for the discussion of sensitive topics. Indeed, the development of the role of the school nurse may make an important contribution to the future well-being of children. Their contact with school children may allow them to promote safe sexual behaviour in the wake of the HIV virus as well as other healthy behaviours. School nurses also have an important role in the detection and prevention of child abuse – their participation in programmes to encourage self-assertion may help reduce the incidence of sexual abuse and experimental drug and solvent use.

A review of support for children and their families has revealed, however, that the end of statutory school life marks the beginning of no support for some young people. As one young person said:

> I'd no back-up, no support, no social workers, nobody visited me, none of that; all seemed to go at one time. Never heard no more ... everything just dropped.
>
> (Stein and Carey, 1986)

The difficulties of children leaving care cannot be underestimated, indeed, it seems about two-thirds are expected to make a physical move at this critical time. In answer to the needs of this special group, a number of projects have been established to assist young people at the time of leaving care, for example, the Leeds Leaving Care Scheme, which is jointly funded by Barnardos and Leeds Social Services Department.

The importance of good support during school life becomes apparent when the employment prospects for different school-leavers are examined. The possession of no graded qualifications leaves children much more vulnerable in the labour market, so that long-term unemployment becomes a prospect for a large number – youth and inner city life is the subject of the following chapter.

CONCLUSION

The evidence appears to suggest that children from inner cities are particularly vulnerable. The educational needs of inner city school children appear to be greater than those of their contemporaries outside the city and, further, it appears that the needs of teaching staff need addressing. The full potential of the school health service has yet to be realized, however, suggestions were made for areas of development in school nursing practice. Changes in health needs among school children pose a challenge to professional workers, in particular, it appears that certain children do not receive the support and guidance they need as they grow up.

REFERENCES

Addy D. P. (1985). Talking points in child abuse. *British Medical Journal*, **290**, 259–60.

Andersen H. R. *et al* (1986). Recent trends in mortality associated with abuse of volatile substances in the U.K. *British Medical Journal*, **293**, 1472–3.

Belsen W. A. (1975). *Juvenile Theft: the causal factors*. London: Harper Row.

Berg I. (1985). The management of truancy. *Journal of Child Psychology and Psychiatry*, (**26**) 3, 325–31.

Black D. (1986). Schoolgirl mothers. *British Medical Journal*, **293**, 25 October, 1047.

British Medical Journal (1985). Solvent abuse (Editorial). *British Medical Journal*, **290**, 12 January, 94.

Cameron J. (1985). Solvent abuse in Glasgow. *Nursing Mirror*, 15 May, 25–6.

Davie R., Butler N. and Goldstein (1972). *From Birth to Seven*. London: Longman.

Department of Education and Science (1980). *Report by the HMI on Educational Provision by the Inner London Education Authority*. London: DES.

Department of Health and Social Security (1976). *Fit for the Future*. Report of the Committee on Child Health Services (Chairman: Professor S. D. M. Court). London: Her Majesty's Stationery Office.

Dobbs J. and Marsh A. (1985). *Smoking among Secondary School Children in 1984*. London: Her Majesty's Stationery Office.

Essen J. and Ghodsian M. (1983). Children of immigrants: school performance; part of Chapter 3: Immigrants, in Fogelman K. (ed.) *Growing Up in Great Britain*. London: Macmillan.

Essen J. and Wedge P. (1982). *Continuities in Childhood Disadvantage*. London: Heinemann Educational.

Family Service Units (1982). *Eneuresis in School Children*. London: Family Service Units.

Field F. (ed.) (1977). *Education and the Urban Crisis*. London: Routledge and Kegan Paul.

Fogelman K. (ed.) (1976). *Britain's Sixteen Year Olds*. London: National Children's Bureau.

Havard J. (1986). Drunken driving among the young. *British Medical Journal*, **293**, 774.

Hill P. (1983a). Children who refuse to go to school. Part 1. *Maternal and Child Health*, 8, (**2**), 58–65.

Hill P. (1983b). Children who refuse to go to school. Part 2. *Maternal and Child Health*, 8, (**3**), 118–20.

Hoghughi M. (1983). *The Delinquent: Directions for Social Control*. London: Burnett Books and Hutchinson.

McClure G. M. G. (1984). Recent trends in suicide among the young. *British Journal of Psychiatry*, **144**, 134–8.

McKerlie L., Hodgson A., McCulloch K. and MacDonald A. (1983). Solvent abuse. *Nursing Mirror*, 14 December. Supplement i–iv.

OPCS (1986a). *General Household Survey 1984*. London: Her Majesty's Stationery Office.

OPCS (1986b). *Social Trends*. **16**. London: Her Majesty's Stationery Office.

Petrie P. and Logan P. (1986). *After School and in the Holidays: the responsibility for looking after school children*. London: Thomas Coram Research Unit.

Plant M. A., Peck D. F. and Samuel E. (1985). *Alcohol, Drugs and School Leavers*. London: Tavistock.

Porter R. (ed.) (1984). *Child Sexual Abuse within the Family*. London: Tavistock.

Reid D. (1985). Prevention of smoking among school children: recommendations for policy development. *Health Education Journal*, **44** (1), 3–12.

Richardson K., Ghodsian M. and Gorbach P. (1983). The association between school variables and attainment in a national sample of 16-year-olds. Part of Chapter 12: Other School Characteristics, in Fogelman K. (ed.) *Growing Up in Great Britain*. London: Macmillan.

Rona R. J. and Chinn S. (1984). The National Study of Health and Growth: nutritional surveillance of primary school children from 1972–1981 with special reference to unemployment and social class. *Annals of Human Biology*, **11** (i), 17–28.

Rutter M. L. (ed.) (1976). *The Child, His Family and the Community*. Chichester: John Wiley.

Rutter M. L., Yule B., Quinton D., Rowlands O., Yule W. and Berger M. (1975). Attainment and adjustment in two geographical areas III: some factors accounting for area differences. *British Journal of Psychiatry*, **126**, 520–33.

Rutter M. and Madge N. (1976). *Cycles of Disadvantage*. London: Heinemann Educational.

Smith G. and Fellner I. (1985). Improving the uptake. *Nursing Times. Community Outlook*. June 46–51.

Stark O., Peckham C. S. and Ades A. (1986). Weights of British and French children. Letter. *Lancet* **1**, 8485, 12 April, 862.

Stein M. and Carey K. (1986). *Leaving Care*. Oxford: Basil Blackwell.

Tibbenham A. (1983). Housing and truancy. Part of Chapter 2: Housing, in Fogelman K. (ed.) *Growing Up in Great Britain*. London: Macmillan.

Todd G. E. and Dodd T. (1985). *Children's Dental Health in the U.K. 1983*. London: Her Majesty's Stationery Office.

Wedge P. and Essen J. (1982). *Children in Adversity*. London: Pan.

Wild N. J. (1986). Sexual abuse of children in Leeds. *British Medical Journal*, **292**, 1113–16.

Williams S., Forbes J. F., McIlwaine G. M. and Rosenberg K. (1987). Poverty and teenage pregnancy. *British Medical Journal*, **294**, 3 January, 20–1.

USEFUL ADDRESSES

Institute for the Study of Drug Dependence,
1–4 Hatton Place, London, EC1N 8ND
Telephone: 01-430 1991

National Out of School Alliance,
Oxford House, Derbyshire Street, London E2
Telephone: 01-739 4787

4

Youth

GILLIAN CHAPMAN

INTRODUCTION

There is a range of theoretical models and related empirical research with which to describe the life experiences of young people. Mainly drawn from psychology, sociology, and the biomedical sciences the literature includes epidemiological and education research. In this chapter the experience of young people living in the inner city will be described with reference to this theoretical and empirical material. Particular attention will be paid to the problems of unemployment, delinquency, running away and drug abuse. A description of the provisions available to this age group together with an account of innovative projects and facilities addressing the problem areas mentioned above are provided.

THEORETICAL APPROACHES TO YOUTH

One of the problems associated with the study of young people between the ages of 16 and 20 years is that they do not fit into a single developmental and social category. They are neither wholly children nor completely adults and this ambiguity is reflected in the literature. For example, this age group are referred to as adolescents in the psychological and psychiatric literature and as youth in sociological and educational literature. In contrast, there seems to be no specific discipline associated with the age group in bio-medical discourse. Further, social historians have pointed out that the notion of adolescence had no meaning in pre-industrial Europe where persons were perceived of as either children or adults. They were not subject to the period of dependency, associated with education, characteristic of developed countries in the twentieth century (Gillins, 1974). There are also difficulties in finding material associated specifically with the experiences of young people in the inner city, and much has to be inferred from the literature on the general subject area of inner city life or the life of young people. The approach taken here, therefore, will be to draw from research and theoretical material which is relevant to youth in the inner city, even though it may not directly focus on young people in these areas.

There is agreement about the core physiological, psychological and social developments which occur during adolescence. First, physiological research demonstrates that general body growth (height, weight, proportion and distribution of fat) development of the reproductive system and secondary sexual characteristics leads to a temporary loss of sensory motor coordination and changes in body image (Law, 1985). Problems likely to arise may be associated with differences in the timing of growth and development, the environmental, emotional and socio-economic climate in which the young person grows up, or failure to develop at puberty. Torsion of the testes is, for example, fairly common among boys, and dysmenorrhea or irregular menstruation is fairly common in girls. Other physical problems (which may have a psychogenic root) encountered by young people include anorexia nervosa, some malignancies, sexually transmitted diseases and, most commonly in boys, trauma due to accidents.

Second, psychologists and psychoanalysts have identified changes in cognitive functioning, moral reasoning and a general reorganization of personality as young people identify with peers, separate from parents and establish their own identity (Coleman, 1980; Erikson, 1983). Psychological problems which arise from psychosexual development, separation anxieties and attempts to establish a satisfying adult identity may lead to profound depression or behavioural problems in this age group. Schizophrenic illnesses may also occur at this time.

Third, sociologists have identified the role of culture in mediating the experience of leaving school, finding work and establishing adult social roles. Clearly the attitude of those around them will affect the young person's adaptation to adult life and some common themes can be identified.

The Open University team (OU, 1977) argues that there are

three main approaches in the popular culture to young people. The first, the 'great gap' thesis, stresses the discontinuities between younger and older generations. Differences between the young and the old are emphasized. Youth protest is perceived in terms of a failure of the socialization process (within the family and at school) to transmit social values in the face of economic and social change. Such views are emphasized by the moral panics which from time to time sweep society and the media in response to the delinquent behaviour of a relatively small group of young males — for example, football hooligans (Cohen, 1972). Second, the 'nothing really new' thesis which suggests that the difference between young people and other members of society is more apparent than real, 'a gloss fostered by the media' which disguises the real similarity and continuity of values between generations. Third, a 'selective continuity' thesis which suggests that there are divisions between young and old in some areas but not others and that these are a function of the complexity of industrial society rather than age and generation. An example might be the computer literacy of the young, compared to the computer incompetence of their parents, which relates to technological developments rather than generational differences. The Open University team point out, however, that a common problem of many studies of young people which implicitly use these approaches is that young people are bracketed together as a homogenous group.

Brake (1985), as a result of his studies of youth culture, challenges the idea of a cultural hegemony of youth. Rather, empirical studies seem to demonstrate that young people fall into four main categories none of which are mutually exclusive.

Respectable youth. Concerned with groups of youths who conform to establishment values while adopting some aspects of teenage culture not considered deviant. Here the appropriation of the clothes or fashions of a deviant life style rather than the life style itself are adopted. (In the mid-1980s many young people adopted the fashions of Boy George without adopting his life-style.)

Delinquent youth. Concerned with studies of young adult males from mainly working-class backgrounds who are involved in illegal activities such as theft, vandalism or violence. Female delinquents are usually seen in terms of their sexual 'misbehaviour'. Most empirical studies fall into this group and include the work of sociologists (Hall and Jefferson, 1977) and psychologists (Rutter and Giller, 1983).

Cultural rebels.   Concerns the study of subcultures on the fringes of Bohemian tradition. Examples include studies of hippies and beats (Willis, 1977).

Politically militant youth.   Concerns groups involved in the radical traditions of politics. This might include environmental politics (Greenpeace) or community issues (CND).

Brake's reminder that young people do not belong to a homogenous group has been followed by a reminder by feminist writers that research and theory related to young people has universally concentrated on white males and their experiences and attitudes. Distinct differences between the experience of girls and boys and black and white youth have been identified. In a series of papers edited by McRobbie and Neva (1984) researchers demonstrate that young girls face a persistent set of interactions with boys and society as a whole which reflects general social attitudes towards women; namely, that they be defined by their perceived sexual availability (or lack of it) to men. Thus girls at a time when their male peers are being encouraged to compete and achieve in the academic and work-related fields have to find ways of coping with an undermining of their intellectual identity. Similarly, black male youth (Cash-more and Troyna, 1982) faces racism and social disadvantage, while black female youth faces sexism, racism and social disad-vantage (Lees, 1986). Social disadvantage can also accrue to white working-class young people, who, if male, may adopt values and behaviour associated with an anti-school machismo as a means of coming to terms with and embracing their perceived future role on the factory floor.

The youth subcultures which arise around these differing experiences seem to serve a particular function and are described by Brake (1985). They:

1. Offer a solution to structural problems (class, race, gender) experienced collectively.
2. Offer a culture which includes style, values, ideologies and behaviour which can be used to develop an identity outside that offered at school or work.

3. Provide an alternative social reality based within a young person's own class and culture, mediated by their own neighbourhood experience, and transmitted via the media in the form of pop and fashion.
4. Offer a meaningful life-style during leisure time distinct from the instrumental world of work and school.
5. Offer an individual solution for certain existential dilemmas. For example, football hooliganism offers a way in which subordinate males may express superordinate male values of territoriality, power and so on.

The small-scale studies into youth described above provide an insight into the meaning to young people of the experiences they face. Research in the social survey and epidemiological traditions provide a demography of youth, and this is outlined below.

DEMOGRAPHY OF YOUTH

Nationally and internationally, governments have demonstrated an interest in young people as illustrated by two surveys about their attitudes and activities published in the early 1980s. There is reason to suppose that young people in the inner city will share some of the preoccupations of their peers identified in these surveys. The Organization for Economic Co-operation and Development, which includes nations such as the USA, Japan, Australia, and the United Kingdom commissioned a review of the views of the young. This seemed motivated by a desire to establish the extent to which the economic recession had undermined their loyalty to the State. Their findings make fascinating reading (OECD, 1983).

The researchers predicted that by the mid-1980s about 17% of the population of member countries (with some variations) would be young people between 15 and 24 years. Most would be at school, but by 19 years many would be unemployed (25% in the United Kingdom and France). In the United States of America, United Kingdom and Australia 50% of black youngsters would be unemployed. These figures are largely supported by more recent data; more fascinating perhaps was their analysis of attitudes.

The attitudes of the young to key areas of the family, the

state, adult life and work shared common patterns across nations. Most young people in all nations reviewed were positive about family life and lived at home. The clashes which occurred with parents seemed to be concerned with specific behaviour related to clothes, friends, and general outlook on life. Most young people felt that their parents tried to understand them but could not. Similarly most of the young felt patriotic towards their country (95% of American, 90% Australian and 83% of English youth). However, they held themselves apart from the country's political processes, or were dissatisfied about the way things were done. The dissatisfactions most commonly expressed were concerned with destruction of the environment and inequalities in social welfare derived from wealth or family background. The feeling that hard work was not recognized completed this list. Such dissatisfactions led, not to revolution, but legal protests, strikes and petitions. The riots in the inner city in England in the early 1980s were perhaps an exception to this rule.

The ambitions for adult life held by the sample seemed centred on the notion to 'live as I like' which, while not stressing wealth, did emphasize the importance of family life and social and economic success. From a third to a half of young people felt education was the key to social advancement. There was no rejection of the work ethic and young people seemed to have a realistic if pessimistic view of their work chances. This may be why at least 50% of the sample found more satisfaction outside their work environment.

Overall the OECD report commented that the evidence suggested young people were trapped between a past they ignore and a future no one could forecast with any certainty. Changes in economic conditions and opportunities and prospects for young people had not led to political revolt but adaptation. One way of adapting seems to have been the adoption of alternative life-styles, as the rising rates of drug addiction, juvenile crime and alcohol consumption demonstrate. It is possible that the life style of the so-called 'football hooligan' is yet another way of adapting to poor prospects. Some of these problem areas will be discussed fully later, here it is worth specifically examining the experience of youth in Great Britain.

The Department of Education and Science (DES, 1983) commissioned a survey of young people's attitudes and activities in the early 1980s, and the provisions available for them.

A detailed description was obtained of young people's

thoughts about themselves and their relationships to others. The
survey revealed many sex, race and social differences. Boys, for
example, were more likely to say positive things about themselves than girls, who were less confident in terms of their
perceived personal characteristics. West Indians (72%) and
Asians (63%) were more likely to report having lots of friends
than Caucasians (49%), although parents in these groups tended
to be less likely to approve of opposite sex relationships.

The young people's use of leisure time also proved of interest,
and seemed to involve a range of activities; those specifically
designed for them, and those available to other members of the
community. The findings were as follows:

Sports.   64% of the sample said they were involved in sporting
activity, and nearly half of those attended a sports centre.

Clubs and associations.   About one-third had attended a youth
club and still attended, 16% had belonged to school clubs, 8% of
the sample had belonged to Girl Guides or Boy Scouts.

Pubs, discos, cinema.   Young people reported wishing to be
involved in community entertainment available to the adult
population but lack of money often limited regular attendance.
An exception to this was going to the pub; 46% of the older
members of the sample went to the pub, 30% to discos and 56%
to the cinema.

Street life.   The street life of adolescents (as perhaps for adults)
tends to happen by default rather than design and consisted of
certain patterns of activity associated with going out with
friends. Forty-four per cent of the sample went window shopping, 43% went to music shops and a small proportion just
'messed about in shops'. Just over a third biked around and just
under a third drove around in a car. Going to cafés and chippies
was fairly popular (43%), and 21% of the sample went to
amusement arcades. A quarter of the sample just 'hang about in
the street'. Apparently community centres were rarely used.
Surprisingly, as many as 26% of the sample had attended a
church, synagogue, or temple event fairly recently.

Alcohol and drugs.   In keeping with reports of regular pub
attendance 55% of the sample said they drank occasionally, 20%

regularly. Most of the drinking seems to occur in pubs or at home with parents, but a fair number (30% and 37%) reported drinking in clubs or at friends' homes. The DES team state that the young people had views about the desirability of drinking. They seemed aware of the possible negative effects of drinking, a large proportion (91%, 84%, 88%) saying it could lead to fights, police trouble, or feeling sick respectively. The positive elements seemed associated with sociability and reduction of stress and anxiety. There was also considerable awareness of types of drug abuse. They knew about glue-sniffing (94%), marijuana (79%) and heroin (72%), less than 38% knew about uppers, downers, speed and cocaine. Just over half of the young people 'knew of' someone who had abused drugs, of these 39% concerned marijuana, 32% glue-sniffing, and only 10% and 8% heroin and cocaine respectively. More than two-thirds (67%) rejected the use of drugs completely, and a quarter (25%) approved partially.

The findings of the national and international surveys mentioned above provide a substantive insight into the subtlety and sophistication of young peoples' attitudes towards the social and economic world in which they find themselves and over which they have little power. It is less easy to discover how these experiences are transformed by the experience of inner city life in Great Britain. In an attempt to do this a general account of family life in the inner city will be discussed in the next section, together with some theories put forward to explain the social disadvantage experienced by young people and their families in this setting.

SOCIAL DEMOGRAPHY OF THE INNER CITY

It is safe to assume that young people in the inner city would share some of the preoccupations of young people in the general culture. However, the life experiences of people in the inner city do differ from their contemporaries in rural and urban environments. The purpose of this section is to explore some of those differences. It is important to note at the outset, however, that information about inner city life is mostly concerned with the impact on families rather than on young people.

The identification of the inner city, as a focus of attention for social reform, has a long history in social science literature.

It started with the work of individuals like Chadwick and Rowntree in the early part of the twentieth century when the links between poverty and town life were first established. Preoccupations with family life (within which most young people reside) in the inner city is concerned with compassion for disadvantage and fear of social disorder (Quinton, 1982). Many studies have demonstrated that inner city areas tend to be populated by families of low social status (working class, single parents, ethnic minorities) in overcrowded conditions of poor quality and deteriorating housing. In these areas there also tend to be high rates of juvenile delinquency, crime, alcoholism, psychiatric disorder, suicide, parasuicide, illegitimate births, divorce, and mental hospital admissions (Rutter and Giller, 1983). Explanations of this and the stereotype of inner city life these rates imply is a contested and controversial area. Quinton (1982) points out that families with problems who reside in inner city areas are not necessarily problem families and that other urban environments (like housing estates) have similar experiences. However, the catalogue of social problems the rates reflect, and the social processes which produce them, are not well understood. Similarly the problems of social disadvantage generally and its explanation are not agreed (Hamnett et al, 1976). There are series of cycles of deprivation and disadvantage in urban society. Low wages, poverty, irregular wages and unemployment are associated with poor accommodation, poor physical and environmental conditions and overcrowding. These, in turn, are linked to strain, physical ill-health and stress. Overall, this environment produces a poor educational background for children and young people who, under-achieving at school, fail to develop the required occupational skills required to earn high wages. Upward social mobility becomes less likely and the cycle of deprivation is thus complete. The problem is, however, that while such cycles of disadvantage have a spatial location (e.g. the inner city) it does not mean they have a spatial cause amenable to spatial interventions. Slum clearance in the 1960s and 1970s did not mean that social disadvantage disappeared but rather it was relocated to the urban and suburban housing estates. It is probable, as in London's Docklands, that when money is put into the inner city areas the poor get pushed out. For the purposes of planning provisions for young people in the inner city it is vital to know therefore whether deprivation attaches to a particular individual or a particular locality. It is the explanatory theories in this area which are the subject of political controversy. The above authors cite five types of explanation of social disadvantage:

1. *Culture of poverty.*   Here it is suggested that certain groups in society (working class, single parents, immigrants, for example) exhibit a form of social pathology. They are, in short, socially maladaptive. It is thought that social incompetence leads to poverty, and therefore the proper method of intervention is to provide social education and supportive social work. Key concept: *Poverty.*

2. *Cycle of deprivation.*   Here the family or individual is seen as being psychologically handicapped. It is the impoverished interpersonal relationships between people which lead to deprivation. It is thought that psychological deprivation is transmitted intergenerationally. Methods of help are concerned with providing counselling, supportive social work, or self-help groups. Key concept: *Deprivation.*

3. *Institutional malfunction.*   Here it is the failures at bureaucratic level which are stressed. Town planning, management, and administration are seen to disadvantage certain groups. The means of resolving this is for more rational social policy and planning. Key concept: *Disadvantage.*

4. *Maldistribution of resources.*   This explanation suggests that unequitable distribution of resources in general leads to the production of a group of people with an underprivileged relationship to the political machine and those in power. (For example, women and blacks.) Reallocation of resources by positive discrimination is suggested. Key concept: *Underprivilege.*

5. *Structural class conflict.*   It is argued that the division of labour and the economic system based on private profit determines the relationship of the working class to political and economic structures. Their position is one of inequality. The way to resolve these problems is the redistribution of power and control through raising of consciousness and political organization. Key concept: *Inequality.*

It should be clear from the above sets of explanations (none of

which are mutually exclusive) why the issue of the causes of
inner city deprivation is a matter of political debate. Clinical
practitioners themselves may espouse any one or more of these
explanations to account for their clients' difficulties. At a practical
level community workers may implicitly recognize and use these
different explanations and interpretations of the social disadvantage problem to guide their actions. An example might be
choosing to refer a young homeless drug addict to local
authority housing departments, a social worker, a general prac-
tioner or self-help group. As far as young people in general are
concerned there does seem to be evidence that family adversity
is linked to psycho-social problems and that inner city areas have
more of both. For example, the National Child Development
Survey (Fogelman, 1983) demonstrated that non-attendance at
school is linked to 'low status, high delinquency areas marked by
a concentration of substandard housing' (p. 74). It is thought that
overcrowded conditions might lead to both poor sleeping habits
and inability to do homework, which, in turn, lead to poor
educational attainment and poor attendance at school. The
schoolchild's experience would tend to produce high truancy
rates, and a set of alienated behaviours which might lead to the
social, economic, and psychological problems of youth unemployment, delinquency, drug addition and running away from
home discussed separately below.

UNEMPLOYMENT

Youth unemployment is an international and national problem.
The 1987 edition of *Social Trends* (Griffin, 1987) showed that at
16 years, 31% of young people were still at school, 14% in
further education, 27% on youth training schemes, 16%
employed and 12% unemployed. By the age of 17 years this
pattern had changed: 19%, 11%, and 11% of young people were
in school, further education and higher education respectively,
48% were employed but 20% unemployed. However, half of all
young black males (who mostly live in inner city areas) were
among the unemployed. Unemployment is a particular problem
for academically less gifted young people, who may remain
unemployed for a considerable time. Of all people unemployed
for over one year 15.8% were young men between the ages of 20
and 24 years and 12% young women of the same age group. Of

all people unemployed from between 6 months and 1 year 14.3%
were young men of between 16 and 19 years. A substantial
proportion of young people, therefore, would experience themselves as having bleak economic prospects. For those living in
inner city areas these prospects must seem particularly disheartening in the sense that hopes of improving their standard of life
through employment are grim. The impact of unemployment in
the inner cities (together with poor housing and police/com-
munity relations) was thought by Lord Scarman to have been at
the heart of inner city riots in the early 1980s. As noted earlier,
lack of employment contributes to a feeling of meaninglessness
which itself may lead to adoption of alternative life-styles
associated with delinquency, crime, vagrancy, and drug-taking.
Indeed, an early study of young working-class males specifically
linked poverty, unemployment and petty crime (Parker, 1974).
Various governments have been mindful of the potential problems posed by unemployed youth. Government provisions to
tackle unemployment have a fairly long history. Home (1986)
notes that during certain periods such as the 1930s, 1970s and
1980s, an 'opinion forming élite' were concerned with the
demoralization associated with male youth unemployment.
There was a fear that enforced leisure might lead to revolution-
ary action. Government schemes to cope with the problem led to
the introduction of Unemployment Centres in 1928, and Junior
Instruction Centres in 1934. These were known as dole colleges
and believed to keep young people off the street. Instructions in
manual dexterity were provided but skills based training, relevant to work and economic life, were not included. The JICs were
similar to the Manpower Services Schemes in the 1970s and
1980s. The Youth Opportunities Programme (YOP) was replaced in the early 1980s by the Youth Training Scheme (YTS)
and each have been criticized, both by young people and
opposition parties, as being either non-relevant, only temporary,
or a means of disguising the unemployment figures.

Schemes aimed at tackling youth unemployment can be
divided into those internal to the school and those external to it.

Dale reports (1986) that the Technical and Vocational Educational Initiative introduced by Mrs Thatcher's Government in
1983, was aimed at restructuring the educational curriculum and
to provide technical and vocational training for less academically
gifted children of between 14 and 18 years. It was argued that
the overacademic stress in schools disadvantaged the already

disadvantaged and was inappropriate for the majority of pupils and inappropriate for the needs of the economy. Young people were said to leave school ignorant if not contemptuous of the economic base of the nation. (A view not supported by the OECD survey mentioned earlier.) The critics of the initiative pointed out that it was potentially divisive as it placed some 14-year-olds into a second-class stream at school from which their life chances would be diminished. Further, there is evidence that different schools interpreted TVEI in a range of ways, leading to a variety of experiences for pupils in this group. Criticisms were also levelled at YTS schemes: some young people felt their labour was being exploited for low pay, without providing skills and experience which could be utilized when they left the scheme (Coffield et al, 1986). Gleeson (1986) seems to suggest that some of these views might be justified. Skills trainers working for the MSC are asked to evaluate trainees in terms, among other things, of their personal cleanliness, loyalty to the work place, use of the telephone, and being helpful. While personal attributes of this type are clearly important, if stressed the impression might be gained that a malleable personality rather than craft skill is the most essential part of getting a job. Overall, it would seem that while training initiatives for young people are welcomed, their success is related to their content and its applicability to the market economy.

The YTS provisions are not the only ones provided by government to aid the unemployment situation, a list of alternative schemes is provided in Table 4., together with projects run by voluntary organizations. Community workers should find this background material of use but, further, more detailed information about these schemes is available from the addresses provided at the end of this chapter.

DELINQUENCY

In their excellent review of delinquency studies Rutter and Giller (1983) point out that delinquency rates vary according to geographical area. Delinquency rates are highest in poor, over-crowded, low social status areas in the cities and large conurbations. They are lowest in the affluent and spacious rural areas. Interpretation of these facts must be undertaken with caution. Rutter and Giller point out that the data are collected where the

Table 4.1 Provisions for Unemployed Youth

Name	Agency	Function/Provision
Youth Training Scheme	TC*	Vocational education/Training work experience. 16 and 17-year-olds
Community industry	TC*	12 months temporary employment. 16–19-year-olds
Employment training	TC*	Average of 6 months employment. Training and placement. Those over 18 years. Preference given to 18–25-year-olds
Enterprise allowance scheme	DOE	£40 per week allowance for those setting up new small business
Job clubs	DOE	Advice/Counselling/Support re job applications if unemployed > 6/12
Job search	Job centres	Financial assistance for travelling expenses for job seekers
Job share	Job centres	Splitting jobs
Job start	Job centres	£20 allowance for 6/12 for those unemployed for 12/12 earning < £80 pw
Opportunities for volunteering	DOH	Voluntary work in Health and Social Services facilities
Voluntary work	Range	See 'Spare Time Share Time' NYB 1986
Voluntary projects programme	TC	Voluntary work/Education while on State Benefit
Restart	Job centres	Counselling for the unemployed

Key: TC = Training Commission
DOE = Department of Employment
DOH = Department of Health
NYB = National Youth Bureau
*Specifically aimed at young people

crime is committed rather than at the address where the offender lives. Thus, delinquency rates may be associated with police practices (SUS laws, for example) or opportunities for crime rather than living in the inner city *per se*. However, as indicated earlier, other social problems like alcoholism, mental disorder and so on are higher in the city. One common explanation for this is that people with problems drift into the city. However, some studies cited by the above authors demonstrate that the delinquency rate fell for groups of families who left London. This indicated that the environment itself rather than the characteristics of the individual predisposes to psycho-social disorder. Delinquency rates within cities, towns, boroughs, and enumeration districts differ, which suggests that an area effect is in operation. For example, some studies demonstrate that particular streets or estates become high delinquency areas. Some theorists have argued that this is a result of the selection processes operated by councils; namely, putting problem families into particular housing estates. Others, taking an ecological perspective, look at the co-relation of high delinquency rates, overcrowding, and poor housing. They suggest that personal overcrowding, and its concomitant psycho-social problems, must be understood from the point of view of the perceptions of residents and those involved in problem estates. The ecology of an area might involve the following processes. Problem families placed in certain estates tend to be large families with several children. Studies have shown that there is a high correlation between vandalism and child density. The physical deterioration, graffiti and damage to the street architecture vandalism entails may lead to stereotyping by neighbouring communities, the police, housing authorities, the media and so on. A greater social distance may arise out of the perceptions created of a problematic environment, which in turn may result in a dynamic of police suspicion of youth, and youth resentment and hostility towards the police. Thus a spiral of mutual hostility and resentment leads to further diminishment of the status of the area.

It is difficult to establish what type of direct intervention health care workers in the community can contribute to the problem of delinquency in inner city areas. Such interventions tend to be largely a matter for the juvenile justice system. Currently health care and other provisions for tackling the problem include counselling and psychotherapy where young people are referred to child-guidance clinics, and custodial and non-custodial care in adolescent units, and attendance centres. Young people convicted of criminal offences may also be supervised by probation officers when on suspended sentences, or at times simply cautioned by the police. Perhaps the community worker's role might best be described as timely recognition of potential problems and referral to appropriate agencies, together with social support for the family concerned.

NON-LEGAL USE OF DRUGS

Drug misuse in this section will be defined as those forms of drug-taking which meet social disapproval. This includes possession, for non-medical use, of drugs under the Misuse of Drugs Act. The drugs concerned therefore include cannabis, LSD, opiates, amphetamines and misuse of solvents.

The Institute for the Study of Drug Dependence review of the surveys and statistics of drug-taking in Britain (1987) provides illuminating insights into the prevalence of drug misuse. They caution the reader with respect to the problems associated with defining and adequately measuring the problem. Different surveys use a range of sample sizes and age groups, some concentrate on national and others on local experiences, while the difficulty of receiving honest replies to surveys associated with potentially illegal acts is well known. Nevertheless the findings make interesting reading.

A national opinion poll in 1982 found that 17% of British youngsters between 15 and 21 years admitted taking cannabis, 4% amphetamines, 3% glues, barbiturates, and LSD and finally 1% heroin or cocaine. (In contrast young people's recreational use of approved substances such as alcohol and tobacco was much higher; about 30% of 16–19-year-olds smoke 11–12 per day, and 34% of boys between the ages of 18 and 24 years defined themselves as heavy drinkers; 43% of girls of the same age group reported they were frequent drinkers.) A survey of schools published by New Society in 1986 reported that 17% of secondary school pupils used cannabis, 6% solvents and 2% heroin. West Indians were slightly less likely to have tried cannabis than their white friends, while Asians registered the lowest 'ever tried' figure for drugs. Some schools seem to be of particularly high risk. For example, one Glasgow boys' school reported a prevalence of solvent misuse in 20–25% of its pupils.

One feature of the 1980s was the growing concern of parents, the community and government about the youth of current drug-abusers. It contrasts with the experience of the 1970s where studies of students in colleges demonstrated that about one-third reported having tried cannabis but practically none heroin or cocaine. The ISDD suggest that this figure too has remained fairly constant; in 1978 nearly 30% of students had tried cannabis, 6% LSD and cocaine but practically none heroin.

Drug-abuse indicator studies seem to suggest that problematic drug-taking is worse in the cities. In two Inner London boroughs in 1983 over 14 per 1000 of the population aged between 16 and 44 years used opiates on a daily or nearly daily basis. In contrast Brighton Health Authority produced an annual prevalence rate of 1.5 known opiate users per 1000 population aged between 15 and 35 years. A Health Education Council survey of heroin use among young people seemed to confirm that trend; that heroin use was thought to be particularly high in areas of high unemployment and social deprivation. It is certainly the case that official statistics demonstrate an increase in the number of narcotic drug addicts notified to the Home Office between 1976 and 1985. (Totals 3474 to 14 688.) There seems to have been a particular increase in notified drug addicts among young people. In 1976, 269 people under 21 were notified, by 1985 this figure had risen to 2065. Similarly, the number of newly notified addicts under 21 years increased from 162 in 1976 to 1531 in 1985. By far the biggest increase in type of drug addiction reported during the period was heroin. In 1976, 912 heroin addicts were reported, in 1985 8089.

Not surprisingly, given the increase in numbers of addicts being notified, there has been a concomitant increase in persons found guilty of or cautioned about a drug offence. In 1976, 171 youngsters under 17 years, and 3273 young people between 17 and 20 years were reported by the police. By 1985 826 under 17 years and 6737 between 17 and 20 years were reported by the police. The only optimistic note in the figures was perhaps that police in Scotland reported a reduction in the amount of solvent abuse between 1981 and 1984 (from 3312 to 1192). Overall, then, however problematic the drug statistics, there does seem to have been an increase in drug misuse among young people, leading to an increase in crime. Drug-abuse seems particularly linked to social deprivation and unemployment. The questions to be answered are therefore, why do young people take drugs, and what types of interventions might be helpful in ameliorating the problem?

The Scottish Health Education Group (1986) provide a useful guide to misuse of drugs by young people. They point out that in a 1984 survey of adults and young people about social problems in Scotland, 83% of the sample placed unemployment high on the agenda, 68% drug misuse and 67% glue-sniffing. Parents particularly reported anxiety related to media coverage of the problems associated with drug-abuse and its life-style. Not only the increased risk of AIDS but the effect of law-breaking on the young person's life chances worried the sample. The concern about the spread of the HIV virus among drug-abusers who share needles was emphasized in the Health Education Campaign of 1986/1987. Indeed many workers in the field believed that the provision of free needles to registered addicts would be the single most important provision for this group. Certainly the risk of AIDS seems to be the single most vital message community workers should communicate to young people abusing drugs.

The Scottish Health Education Group (SHEG) believe that the commonest reason for young people using drugs is a mixture of curiosity and pleasure enhanced or encouraged by the approval of their peers. They acknowledge that illicit drugs may be used to relieve stress or to solve problems. Mostly, however, use is casual and seems to be a gesture of rebellion rather than a reflection of profound stress. The availability of the drug also plays a part in the process, which might explain why drug misuse is higher in the cities. The group point out that those people who become deeply involved in the misuse of drugs are unusual for a number of reasons. The most important is that they usually have little stake in the workaday world and may be estranged from their families. For such individuals the drug scene offers a sense of security, purpose and excitement missing in their immediate environment. It is to the 'scene' these people become attached as it produces meaning and a general identity upon which the young person can plan his day.

The fact that the life-style attached to drug-taking is as important to the drug-abuser as the addictive properties of the drug itself, has become increasingly recognized by agencies concerned with ameliorating the problem. It has been found that many young people may experiment with drugs for a while and then drop them or greatly reduce their use. A ten-year follow-up study of London clinics cited by SHEG concluded that of heroin users 38% spontaneously stopped altogether, 38% continued but at a reduced level, and 15% died. There are two comments to make about these figures. The first is that the death rate for a group of young people is high, the second that a sizeable proportion of drug-users seem to have difficulty in giving up. It is perhaps for this last group which provisions are designed. Overall, there are many voluntary agencies and statutory organizations which take an interest in the problem. This is in part because there is little agreement about whether drug addiction is mainly a medical, social or economic problem. One consequence of this is that there is a range of services available, each offering something slightly different. The majority of drug-abusers do not come into contact with health service personnel unless as a consequence of the toxic effects of drugs, or because a relative is concerned about them. The advice given by SHEG is that when young people do come into contact with the health service the following principles should be understood. (1) A broad social perspective should be used to plan care. (2) Drug centred approaches will not succeed without assessment of psychological, social and economic needs of the drug user. (3) Most individuals seen will be multiple drug misusers. (4) An individual's susceptibility to treatment fluctuates over time, consequently sensitivity is required to assess the optimal moment for intervention. (5) Prevention and early detection strategies are better than curative strategies. (6) Doctors' attitudes to prescribing mind altering drugs effect general cultural attitudes to drug-abuse. Examples of types of service available for drug-abusers are listed in Table 4.

HOMELESSNESS AND VAGRANCY

Adult vagrancy and homelessness seems to be linked to alcoholism and unemployment, but homelessness in young people seems to have a different set of causes. In an interesting review of the problems of identifying and measuring the phenomenon of runaways and street children De'Arth (1987) notes that historically governments have always been concerned about this problem. In the 1870s and 1880s the major child voluntary organizations were set up to cater for destitute waifs and strays. Destitute children were exposed to disease and malnutrition, violence, exploitation and prostitution in the past just as today.

Table 4.2   Provisions for Drug-abusers

Agency	Service
General Practitioner	Health education, detection and diagnoses, physical assessment, detoxification programmes, counselling, referral
Community Nursing Services	Recognition, detection, health education – Families, Individuals, School. Self-help groups, counselling, referral to GP
General Hospital Services	Emergencies/Crises. Assessment/Risk of physical side-effects. Referral to specialists
Specialists services	Assessment, health screening, detoxification, rehabilitation
Social Work Departments	Assessment, counselling, referral, family support therapy
Voluntary Agencies	Self-help, relative support, advice, counselling information/education, day centres, residential rehabilitation*

*Range of organisations; see SHEG, 1986 (SHEG = Scottish Health Education Group).

Runaway children today are also likely to be involved in begging and shoplifting. De'Arth cites the Independent Commission on International Humanitarian Issues' definition of a runaway or street child as 'any minor for whom the street has become his or her habitual abode and who is without adequate protection'. UNICEF estimate the global figure of such children and young people to be 30 million. However, adequate measurement is problematic because street youth includes delinquents, latch-key children, child labourers, drop-outs and maladjusted children. Each of these groups comes under the scrutiny of a different agency, the juvenile justice system, social service departments, and the health care services, each of which collect their own statistics and none of which are directly comparable. In the Netherlands it is estimated that 25,000 young children run away in each year. Their system of classification is of interest as it deals with reasons for running away:

Seeking independence: A response to family repression.
Running from problems: A response to family stress, school or unemployment.

Fun seekers: Runaways of a few days searching for the 'bright lights of the city'.

Running from public institutions: Children in care who rejoin family.

Running from stress treatment: Children in long-term care running from relationships.

In the United Kingdom no similar method of classification exists, and there is no coordinated policy for youth that might make the collection of statistics and identification of needs more possible. De'Arth provides a useful outline of terms used in the United Kingdom, and it will be seen how unhelpful these are in the planning of care for this group.

Missing children: Those who disappear, including runaways, abducted and kidnapped children.

Absconders: Those absent from the address of residence by force of law (children's homes, foster homes, hospitals).

Homeless: No fixed abode or permanent accommodation.

Rootless drifters: Those who leave home to seek jobs in London, or seasonal work on the coast. Those who move from place to place living in squats, the streets, the beach.

There are some figures available for the United Kingdom. The Metropolitan Police estimated that there were 869 children missing in the capital in 1985.

In contrast, a Children's Society Survey of twenty-seven chief constables indicated that 42 966 young people were missing during 1985. The Children's Society estimated that on a national basis this figure would rise to 75 000–85 000 young people each year. De'Arth cites the Under Secretary for Health and Social Security for stating that the existing figures were unreliable and that 'appropriate help should be available in London and all our major cities for children who run away or are reported missing' (p. ii). Services for this group are patchy and offered by a range of organizations listed in Table 4. Workers who are used to dealing with young people in this situation stress, however, that given the reasons for running away in the first place, confidentiality and a temporary safe haven are a necessity. One such provision is the Central London Teenage Project run by the Children's Society and described below.

Brown and Mercer (1987) describe the origins and objectives of the project which arose out of the increasing awareness by the

Table 4.3 Provisions for Homeless Youth

Agency	Service
Housing Advice Switchboard	Information
Centrepoint	Information, advice, emergency
Soho Project	night shelter, temporary
Alone in London	accommodation
Message Home: Mothers' Union	Telephone links with parents
Family Network: National Children's Home	Telephone links with parents
Walk-in Clinics	Counselling and advice on family problems

child-care agencies of the problem of young runaways in Camden and Westminster. The Children's Society together with Alone in London Service, Centrepoint, Soho Project and Westminster Social Services Department met and discussed the problem of young people who, having been identified as runaways and sent home, returned to London regularly. It was agreed that young people under 17 years, or in local authority care, who leave home or care of their own accord but without agreement, are forced to leave home, or have been missing for one or more nights, required their own facilities. It was thought that such a facility should be managed by a steering group which included the above agencies and could offer a confidential service in which the youngster would have time to work out his reasons for running away, the consequences, and the options available to him in the future. In order to do this it was vital that the young person felt that the environment was a safe haven from which he could not be removed. It was therefore agreed that if a young person arrived at the project the social worker, police and parents would be informed that he was safe, but only the referring agency would know the address of the house.

A safe house based on these principles was subsequently set up for twelve young people under 17 years of age (or if in care up to 19 years). Its terms of reference were (and are) to assess the needs of the young person and investigate the circumstances of their running away in conjunction with parents or other agencies. The young person is counselled and offered advice, current methods of treatment are evaluated, and alternatives sought if appropriate and possible. Following this the young person is returned to his own home area as quickly as possible. Newman (1987) undertook a follow-up study of the 271 young people seen in the first year of the project. He found that 62% of the young people ran from their families, and 37% from the local authority. Most stayed up to three days, although exceptionally one stayed for three months. Longer stays were accounted for by young people waiting for long-term accommodation. The reasons for running away were overwhelmingly given as poor communications at home, resulting in rows and arguments, parental violence or drunkenness, or problems related to school. Newman reports that 17% of all the youngsters had been sexually abused at some time (25% of girls, 8% of boys). Just over 40% of the sexually abused young women had been raped, 18% were sexually abused by their father and 18% by another male relative. Boys were sexually abused by older men. On following up these young people 74% were found to be back at home, 19% away from home and 7% could not be contacted. A positive sign for the project was that three months after staying at the project most young people reported it as being helpful and safe, with an understanding staff and friendly atmosphere. The success of the project is not, however, unqualified; social workers with their statutory duty to care for young people at risk are reported as being most uncomfortable with the confidentiality rule, embodied in this philosophy.

CONCLUSION

In this chapter the experience of young people, as reflected in a variety of theoretical and empirical studies, has been described. It was noted that young people are involved in a series of overlapping changes. The first, biological changes are associated with general body growth and development of sexual characteristics. These changes involve personal and social adjustments each of which may give rise to health problems. Second, psychological changes are associated with the formation of adult sexual and social identity, separation from home and parents and identification with peers. Further, development of moral reasoning highlights the young person's idealism and disappointment with the establishment world of his parents. Psychological troubles which affect adolescents during this period may include depression or anorexia nervosa. The third, social changes, are concerned with the transition from childhood to adult culture via a series of youth cultures which mediate the social experience of young people. Social troubles which may affect young people during this period are concerned with societal disapproval of alternative life-styles. The examples provided in this chapter include delinquency, running away, and drug-abuse. Unemployment is seen not as an alternative life-style, chosen by the young, but one imposed by the socio-economic conditions of the 1980s. Similarly, troubles associated with the socio-economic experiences of young women and blacks are seen as a function of social structures, attitudes and values rather than personal choice.

Developmental experiences of the young described above were set in the context of studies which describe their thoughts and beliefs about life. Certain patterns of thought seemed very similar throughout the developed world, young people apparently valuing much the same things as their parents; for example, family life, education, social activities and work. However, they seemed dispirited about their own life chances. It was argued that young people in the inner city would share some of the preoccupations described above, but mediated by the harsh social, economic and physical environment in which they grew up and live. Research studies which identify these harsh living conditions and social disadvantage in inner city areas were described, and some competing explanations of social disadvantage and its impact on individuals outlined. The association between inner city areas and high rates of delinquency, drug-taking, unemployment and running away were discussed.

An exploration of some of the reasons which lie behind these problems was followed by a brief account of the provisions and facilities available to these client groups. The emphasis behind the chapter has been to provide the community worker with the knowledge and information which might inform/guide his/her actions when dealing with young people in inner city areas.

REFERENCES

Brake M. (1985). *Comparative Youth Culture: The Sociology of Youth Cultures and Youth Sub-cultures in America, Britain and Canada*. London: Routledge and Kegan Paul.

Brown G. and Mercer B. (1987). A safe house amid turmoil and danger. *Community Care*. 26 Feb. iv–v.

Cashmore E. and Troyna B. (eds) (1982). *Black Youth in Crisis*. London: George Allen & Unwin.

Coffield E., Borril C. and Marshall S. (1986). *Growing Up at the Margins*. Milton Keynes: Open University.

Cohen S. (1973). *Folk Devils and Moral Panics*. London. Paladin.

Coleman J. C. (1980). *The Nature of Adolescence*. London: Methuen.

Dale R. (1986). Examining the gift horse's teeth: A tentative analysis of TVEI, in Walker S. and Barton L. (eds). *Youth, Unemployment and Schooling*. Milton Keynes: Open University.

De'Arth E. (1987). Ordinary children – lonely and frightened. *Community Care*. 26 Feb. i–iii.

Department of Education and Science (1983). *Young People in the 80's: A survey*. London: HMSO.

Erikson E. (1983). *Identity, Youth and Crises*. London: Faber & Faber.

Fogelman K. (ed.) (1983). *Growing Up in Great Britain*. London: Macmillan.

Gleeson D. (1986). Further education, free enterprise and the curriculum, in Walker S. and Barton L. (eds): *Youth, Unemployment and Schooling*. Milton Keynes: Open University.

Griffin T. (ed.) (1987). *Social Trends*, **17**. C.S.O. London: HMSO.

Hall S. and Jefferson T. (eds) (1977). *Resistance Through Rituals: Youth Subcultures in Post-War Britain*. London: Hutchinson.

Hamnett C. (1976). *Multiple Deprivation and the Inner City*. Unit 5. D302. Milton Keynes: Open University.

Home J. (1976). Continuity and change in the state regulation and schooling of unemployed youth, in Walker S. and Barton L. (eds): *Youth, Unemployment and Schooling*. Milton Keynes: Open University.

Institute for the Study of Drug Dependence (1987). *Surveys and Statistics on Drug Taking in Britain*. London: ISDD.

Law C. (1985). Physiological changes in adolescence. *Nursing* **2**, 85 (4), 1173–7.

Lees S. (1986). *Losing Out: Sexuality and Adolescent Girls*. London: Hutchinson.

McRobbie A. and Neva M. (1984). *Gender and Generation*. London: Macmillan.

Newman C. (1987). Statistics of survival. *Community Care*, 26 Feb., vi. Organisation for Economic Co-operation and Development (1983). *Education and Work. The Views of Young People*. London: Centre for Educational Research and Innovation.

Parker H. J. (1974). *View from the Boys*. London: David and Charles.

Quinton D. (1982). Family life in the inner city: myth and reality, in Blowers A. (ed.): *Urban Change and Conflict*. London: Harper & Row.

Rutter M. and Giller H. (1983). *Juvenile Delinquency: Trends and Perspectives*. Harmondsworth: Penguin.

Scottish Health Education Group (1986). *Drugs and Young People in Scotland*. Edinburgh: SHEG.

Willis P. (1977). The cultural meaning of drug use, in Hall S. and Jefferson T. (eds): *Resistance Through Rituals: Youth Subcultures in Post-War Britain*. London: Hutchinson.

Woods P. (1977). Youth Generations and Social Class. Part of *Schooling and Society*, E202, 27–8. Milton Keynes: Open University.

USEFUL ADDRESSES

National Youth Bureau
17–23 Albion Street, Leicester LE1 6GD

Institute for the Study of Drug Dependence
1–4 Hatton Place (off St Cross Street), London EC1N 8ND

5

Family Life

JULIAN HILLMAN

INTRODUCTION

There are no hazard warning signs on the street, suggesting you
are now passing into an inner city area, although the type and
state of the housing, the quality of the shops and the dress and
demeanour of the people almost constitute giving formal notice.
Nor do the children in the schools have completely different
sorts of lessons, although we will discover later on how their
educational achievement is often limited by their socio-economic
situation. Yet most of us have a vague unease about parts of our
cities and do not want to live in their large tower block estates
and crumbling houses, send our children to their ageing Victor-
ian schools or walk their streets, especially at night. We have
heard about American cities and when we can bear to think about
it we are afraid. Many more people live and die on the streets of
New York than London.

The danger of a chapter like this is that it may contribute to a
process of labelling and stigmatizing certain areas and the
families that live there. We create a subspecies of children and
adults to whom we apply different standards and about whom
we have different attitudes. In this chapter the issue of the
appropriateness of applying different attitudes and standards is
considered. Positive discrimination or affirmative action is necessary but can be misunderstood and the freedom to compete
argument so dear to western thinking can easily persuade us that
only personal attitudes matter. The approach taken here is that
readers are concerned with working with and for their fellow
human beings and that to do this successfully involves understanding the experience of inner city living and the feelings and
attitudes it inculcates in its inhabitants. It follows that if this

chapter is correct and some people live in disabling environments, then fairness suggests they have a right to special help if
they are to participate properly in society.

The setting apart process can become that much easier in the
inner city because a sizeable minority who live there are of Afro-
Caribbean or Indian/Pakistani descent. Some inner city areas
seem to be a microcosm of the peoples of the world, with its
relative wealth and relative political freedom sucking in the
ambitious, the repressed and the dispossessed of other lands. The
indigenous population have not been particularly pleased about
Britain's acknowledgement of its colonial promises and libertar-
ian traditions and the helping professions are only just beginning
to fully appreciate the influence of race and culture if the help
they offer is to be properly utilized. Questions about the best
methods of providing treatment, help or care, and how to be
more receptive to consumer feedback, are still open to research
and debate.

Those who feel they do not have their own inner city
experience to draw on, or need reminding, should buy a copy of
Paul Harrison's (1985) *Inside the Inner City: Life Under the Cutting
Edge*. The book is based on about 500 interviews in 1981/2 with
people living and working in Hackney and is a sequel to his book
Inside the Third World. His work makes us aware of the internal
disparities of wealth as a microcosm of the starker contrasts
between the West and the Third World. *Inside the Inner City* can
be dismissed as an emotional book, but only if one experiences
life as Harrison does, with passion and commitment, can one
really be open to the problems of other people's lives. It is not a
biased book, presenting, for example, police in a realistic and
understandable way and making plain the divisions that deprivation causes – how the poor residents of Hackney destroy and
abuse each other and themselves rather than threatening the
stability of suburban life further out of London. Harrison says he
is concerned with the problems of Hackney and he believes 'the
pathology of a society can be diagnosed from its victims' (p. 12).
The alternative Hackney is always to be found, however it is in
the contrasts and the proportions of winners and losers, that the
lessons are learned.

THE CONTEXT: JOBS COME AND JOBS GO

Proper industrialization began roughly 150 years ago in this country, although its roots lie in the achievements of the inventive engineers of the eighteenth century. Factories and cities grew in places where natural resources and geography could combine to create the ideal site for production. People were sucked into these expanding areas and multiplied there as economics, public health developments and infant mortality allowed. For many people it was never a good life, but it eventually created the large middle class we know today and upward social mobility was a real possibility especially at times of greatest economic expansion. Yet now we are besieged with news about the demise of our inner cities, with the causes and solutions being a source of heated debate. The pinnacle of our world trade leadership is 100 years past and since the last war the centres of heavy industry have moved towards the cheap labour markets of the Third World. There is uncertainty as to whether high technology, financial, insurance, and service industries will continue to support this country's current standard of living. Can the country continue to afford the support it now puts into the inner cities? Can fiscal and financial priorities be rejigged if the national cake is not going to get any bigger?

Automatic Poverty (Jordan, 1981) suggests that technology has meant, and will continue to mean, the replacement of paid workers by sophisticated machinery. Current comparisons with other industrialized nations made as a spur to the United Kingdom working harder are to little avail. We are in a different stage of development in terms of time elapsed since initial industrialization, population growth, wage levels and movement from the land to the factories. Levels of production will be maintained while the numbers employed continue to fall. Public services and welfare agencies may have a role in pointing out to society and their consumers/clients that adjustments in attitudes to the work ethic, social security and the unemployed and their families will be necessary if we are to meet the challenge of the changing economic structure of British society. Whatever the rights and wrongs of the miners' strike, the subsequent job losses in the industry make it plain that the miners' fears were justified. Whether their struggle made the decline more or less severe will remain on the political agenda for some time.

Since the 1977 White Paper, 'Policy for the Inner Cities', the

Department of the Environment has in partnership with local authorities invested money into the inner cities in an attempt to regenerate them. Some commentators regard these sums as insufficient to do this job, others suggest we cannot prop up the edifice of the inner cities by subsidies, it is just throwing money at a problem. With the increase in unemployment, which has been particularly severe in the 1980s, much money has gone into job creation and training. Again there is much debate about value and effectiveness. Can good products and services be created in the small factory/office units the Government has encouraged? Are the right skills available? Can the products and services be got to the people with money in suburbia here and abroad? Schools have been targeted with the provision of educational priority areas, housing improvement areas have been identified and statutory and voluntary social services have been supported. Yet in terms of the macro economic realities it may be that we are running hard to stay still, as flight from the inner cities continues to the urban 'sunshine' belts of South-East England or Cheshire for those who can afford their own house and transport. Economic and fiscal policy, it is argued, supports the middle classes with their mortgage and superannuation tax relief and their company cars. It is convincingly argued that the middle classes do best out of the welfare state (Le Grand, 1982).

Faith in the City, the Report of the Archbishop of Canterbury's Commission on Urban Priority Areas (UPAs) (1985) suggests that 'it is the national decline in the numbers of manual workers in the UPAs that lies at the heart of the problem'. By 1981 there were nearly 2 million fewer manual worker jobs in the United Kingdom than in the early 1970s. The major part of the decline in full-time male manual worker jobs (1.8 million) related closely to the absolute decline in employment in the manufacturing and constructing sectors of the economy (p. 202). The growth of female, frequently part-time, work is of course to be welcomed. However considering the way families are structured, if a man cannot find reasonably paid, full-time employment, then the pressures on all members of the family are considerable, not only in terms of meeting modern basic expectations, but also in declining self-esteem and resultant psychological damage.

In the inner cities many men's prospects of getting back into work are bleak. The problem of unemployment among school-leavers is particularly worrying, with rates around and above 30% recorded in Birmingham, Newcastle, Liverpool and Man-

chester in 1981. The Government is very properly now committed to training schemes for everyone in this age group. However
important Youth Training Schemes become, there are still the
issues of what sort of jobs there will be for youngsters to go into
and whether we can restructure the education, training and
industry of our nation, so that the one-third of the population
whose relative standard of living is dropping can catch up those
of us on whom the sun still shines.

WHY POVERTY, AND WHO DO WE BLAME?

Two issues demand consideration when reflecting on information about poverty. Firstly, how concerned should we be about
the poor inner city family? After all, what used to constitute
riches may now be regarded as poverty and people's expectations and standards are so much higher today, perhaps unrea-
sonably so? Secondly, are the poor not responsible for their own
plight and so why should we be concerned? Could not our
concern be counter-productive and undermine the very thrust for
independence that helps people stand on their own feet?

The contention that poverty has been abolished by the post-
war reforms of the Attlee Government has been hotly argued
and denied since Townsend reopened the debate in the 1960s
(Abel-Smith and Townsend, 1965). Many writers quote Booth's
and Rowntree's seminal poverty survey work in the East End and
York respectively, which helps to link us with the attitudes of the
previous century when both men were collecting their data,
although Rowntree was still at work in the 1930s making a useful
link between the last century and the mid-twentieth century.
Booth defined poverty as the inability to afford the necessities of
life and Rowntree considered the necessities to relate to physical
efficiency. Rowntree's concept of subsistence poverty was based
on the premise that a family

> must never purchase a half penny newspaper or spend a
> penny to buy a ticket for a popular concert. They must write
> no letters to absent children for they cannot afford to pay
> the postage. They must never contribute anything to their
> church or chapel, or give any help to a neighbour which
> costs them money ... the children must have no pocket
> money for dolls, marbles or sweets. The father must smoke
> no tobacco and must drink no beer.
>
> (quoted in Briggs, 1961, p. 38)

More recently Piachaud (1979) has established that supplementary benefits provide only two-thirds of what a very modest household might need to clothe, feed and warm a child; he did, however, include a week at Butlins in his calculations! For working parents, the cost of a child turned out to be twice the level of child benefit. In relation to the question about standards Piachaud says 'there is no such thing as a rational, scientific or objective basis for what a child requires'.

Poor Britain (Mack and Lansley, 1985), based on the commercial television programme Breadline Britain, gives its own detailed consideration to poverty definition and takes the social participation and relative deprivation approach. As Halsey (1981) says, 'What determines behaviour is not actual but felt deprivation.' If a family cannot share in the life of the community then exclusion and stigmatization will occur. People feel different.

Fred Hirsch's (1976) important book *The Social Limits to Growth*, written in the second half of the 1970s when it was clear the post-war economic expansion was over, points out that if everybody increases their standard of living as they did in the 1950s and 1960s then they are likely to be relatively content, but that individualized improvements especially at the expense of public provision can damage social cohesion, an issue which underlies much of what is said in this chapter.

In terms of real poverty the author recommends that readers in doubt work out from the information at the end of this chapter (see Table 5.2) what the Income Support (until April 1988, supplementary benefit) levels for them or their family would be and then consider organizing Christmas on that basis. The point is perhaps honed by watching an evening's commercial television which makes no allowances for how families living on Income Support curtail or control their desires.

As regards attitudes to the poor an EEC Survey in 1976 established that 43% of United Kingdom residents were likely to believe that poverty was attributable to 'laziness and lack of will power' (Mack and Lansley, 1985). By the time 'Breadline Britain' did its survey in 1984, this was down to 22%. In 1976 the EEC also found 16% of the population of Britain saw poverty in terms of injustice, although the figure was 26% in the EEC itself. When 'Breadline Britain' did its survey in 1984, 32% of United Kingdom residents attributed poverty to injustice. Current unemployment levels seem to have changed people's attitudes.

This chapter considers writings that do not suggest that laziness breeds poverty so much as poverty breeds depression and despair. First impressions as a trainee health visitor, GP or social worker from a previously middle-class environment may well suggest that the attitudes of many deprived inner city dwellers are strange and unhelpful to them in their plight. Reflection upon experience suggests that if behaviour is not adaptive, i.e. an appropriate response to the circumstances, then it is quite difficult to formulate a different type of explanation other than one that boils down to indigenous moral failure. In religious terms this might imply more than one's fair share of original sin.

Holman (1978) in his book *Poverty Explanations of Social Deprivation* arrives at what he calls a 'structural adaptive' explanation, i.e. that within the wider economic social and cultural system the poor manage and adapt their behaviour in the way they can — they react to the changing pattern of circumstances they experience — we all do! Holman suggests that 'the poor are constrained to adopt child rearing methods, attitudes to education and work, family behaviour patterns and individual reactions which both further disadvantage their children's development and appear to prove that they are fit for nothing else except poverty' (p. 238). This is not a deterministic approach *per se* as will be seen from the way this chapter develops, nor does it imply that nature or heredity plays no part in how children grow to adulthood.

WHY STAY IN THE INNER CITY? HOUSING AND HOMELESSNESS

Poverty, not choice, is the factor that keeps people in the run-down inner city areas. However, well-to-do people still live in selected parts of the inner cities. In the Royal Borough of Kensington and Chelsea, as you move from Ladbroke Grove to the King's Road, rags and riches can be seen cheek by jowl. Such proximity is the exception rather than the rule and the vast council estates of East and South-East London are more typical. *Faith in the City* argues that it is the large housing estates in the inner ring or on the fringes of the cities that present the most pressing urban problem of the mid-1980s. These estates are stigmatized and only the desperate accept tenancies there. Those estates on the fringe of cities are further dogged by transport problems and lack of facilities. The present Government's policy is based on home ownership and choice, but freedom of choice, says *Faith in the City*, is a 'cruel deception' (p. 231) for those in these large estates.

Investment in public housing has greatly decreased and sale of the public stock (over 650 000) at less than market value has, not surprisingly, been very popular. Incredibly the Government has not wanted to put all of the cash returns into more council accommodation. Such a policy would also have brought much needed jobs to inner city areas.

Although two out of three households are owner occupiers, there are considerable regional variations. The poorer parts of the country are below average with the South-East and South-West well above. This is the case even though house prices are much lower in poorer areas. This obviously has implications for those who might move to the areas with more jobs but are owner occupiers in less economically favoured parts of the country.

In the inner cities much of the traditional housing is pre-First War and crumbling. Rented accommodation is in particularly poor repair and rapidly decreasing (less than 10% of households), as it gives a landlord poor return on capital. Housing Associations have made a relatively small (2% of all households) but significant contribution to acquiring and repairing older property. It is well known that there is great concern about the quality of the post-Second War systems building and equal concern about its effect on people's lives. Streets in the sky are a discredited concept. Stories of demolishing relatively modern but unsafe or uninhabitable blocks are familiar. The experience as a professional helper of visiting the top of a tower block with the wind whistling around the windows and ventilators is that one can feel as isolated up there as on a tor on Dartmoor. Few would choose such isolation as home.

Recent housing policies have massively decreased capital and revenue expenditure on public housing. This means reduction in new public accommodation, higher rents relative to the cost of living and increasing problems about the state of repair of existing housing. Demand for housing has, however, increased.

The sharp end of housing need is those accepted as homeless by local authorities under the Housing (Homeless Persons) Act 1977 (now 1985 Housing Act (Part III)). In 1984, 83 000 households were accepted under the Act. In the six months to 30.9.86, London Boroughs accepted over 15 000 households as homeless. The use of Bed and Breakfast hotels is growing and as SHAC (Conway and Kemp, 1985) points out it is a waste of public money, as better housing could be acquired more economically instead of paying huge sums to hoteliers. There are many other people in hotel type accommodation, not found for them as homeless people, but as single people not eligible under the Act, the only space they can find. In 1982 there were over 84 000 households (97% single people) claiming supplementary benefit in board and lodging type accommodation in Great Britain. It is probable this figure is in the process of doubling, swollen by increased unemployment among the young.

Housing finance is a very complex area. We have already noted large cuts in Government investment in public housing. The *Guardian*'s first leader of 3.12.85 says that council rents have risen by 150% since 1979 – far higher than inflation – so that the majority of councils are now putting money from the council housing account into the general rate fund. In contrast the leader writer notes the cost of mortgage tax relief has risen from £1.1 billion in 1978/9 to an estimated £4.5 billion in 1985/6. In 1985 the *Report of the Enquiry into British Housing*, chaired by the Duke of Edinburgh, recommended recycling of mortgage relief into a broadly based housing allowance aimed at the less well off regardless of their form of tenure. It also recommended an expanded rented sector and agreed with the accepted view that it would take many billions to put the country's housing stock to rights.

By not putting more money into public housing we are re-establishing the link between poverty and inadequate housing. At the time of writing, it is hard to see how the Government's plans to bring more private accommodation into the market by doing away with controls and encouraging council tenants to buy their homes or choose new landlords will, without increased finance, help to house poor families.

WHAT HAPPENS TO CHILDREN LOCKED IN THE INNER CITY?

Disadvantage stemming from poverty does not only manifest itself in poor housing. All facets of life—health, education, work, social and leisure opportunities, even domestic and family life itself, are likely to be adversely affected. For our purposes this is best demonstrated by considering the results of the National Child Development Study, a project monitoring the progress from birth to maturity of all those in England, Scotland and Wales born in one week of March 1958. *Born to Fail?* (Wedge and Prosser, 1973), which sampled the children at 11 years, demonstrated that the social adversities faced by some boys and girls reached into almost every aspect of their health, their family circumstances and their eduational developments. *Children in Adversity* (Wedge and Essen, 1982) looked at the same children when they were 16 and also found a disadvantaged group of children who failed to thrive, mature, grow or achieve as well at school as other children. These children were identified by:

1. Family composition — five or more children under 21 or lack of one parent.
2. Low income — receiving supplementary benefit or on low income and getting free school meals.
3. Poor housing — either more than one and a half persons per room or no hot water supply for the family's exclusive use.

The National Child Development Study report is careful not to say disadvantage is caused by these factors but that there is a direct or indirect link. Many children suffered one or two of these three adversities but the group that *Children in Adversity* identified as 'disadvantaged' suffer all three.

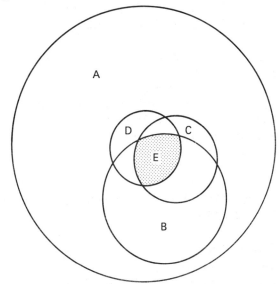

Fig 5.1
*Diagrammatic
identification of
the
Disadvantaged!*

**Fig. 5.1   Adversities Among Children at Age 11 and Again
at 16**

		At age 11 (1969)	At age 16 (1974)
A	No adversities	71%	73%
B	One parent/large family	20%	19%
C	Poorly housed	15%	12%
D	Low income	13%	10%
E	Disadvantaged	4.5%	2.9%

Wedge & Esson, 1982, p. 25.

The improvements suggested by these figures may be accounted for in part by national economic growth and in part by the positional improvements a family with older children may have made relative to the general condition of all families. Wedge and Essen (1982) argue that: 'If our figures applied across the whole range of childhood up to the end of compulsory schooling, there will have been at least half a million children growing up socially disadvantaged in 1974. Given the subsequent national economic difficulties this number could have risen even higher since that time' (p. 27). The Child Poverty Action Group will tell you it has.

THE NORTH/SOUTH DIVIDE

As one might expect, the National Child Development Study survey is clear these disadvantaged children are more numerous further north. Glasgow is particularly highlighted with 10% of Scottish children being disadvantaged at age of 11 or 16 years twice the proportion in England and Wales. Mack and Lansley (1985) suggest that, in 1983, 7 million people lived in families supported by supplementary benefit payments and that by their definitions 'there are 2.6 million people including 1 million children who live in intense poverty: that is about 1 in every 20 people (p. 185). *Poor Britain* also says there is a sharp north/south divide – 'over two-thirds of those in poverty live in Scotland, the north of England and the Midlands while under half the comfortably off live in these areas. The concentration in the northern cities of those in intense poverty is stark. This reflects the massive extent of any inner city decay in conurbations like Merseyside and the sharp impact of the recession in these areas' (p. 189).

LOOKING IN DETAIL AT WHAT AFFECTS
CHILDREN'S DEVELOPMENT

Obviously not all disadvantaged children live in the inner cities, nor do all families in the inner city function in the same way. A study called *Parents and Children in the Inner City* by Wilson and Herbert (1978) highlights the effect socio-economic factors have in child-rearing method, child behaviour and social development and school performance. They took fifty-six families with five or more children living in an area of inner city deprivation in the Midlands and known to the local social services department. They chose families with two parents, not necessarily married or the parent of all the children in the family, and excluded immigrant families apart from Irish to avoid criticism that their findings were affected by racial/cultural factors. They focused on two children in each family: one 3 to 4 years and a school-age boy, and compared them with a control group and a random sample from the same area. In a painstakingly detailed survey they point out how the children were generally seen by their parents in terms of the degree of usefulness or nuisance which they exhibited in family life. Punishment was usually administered indiscriminately to curb noise or conflict without regard for the wrongdoer. The impact of different child rearing patterns on child development was severe. There was evidence of boys in the average range of ability achieving well below the average in reading. The school, and the area in which the school was, they also found influential. Behaviour difficulties in class do increase in relation to the level of social handicap experienced. The sample children get less individual attention, care from siblings rather than parents and of course have few individual possessions. Delinquency and poor classroom adjustment are, they think, related to what they call lack of parental 'chaperonage' (p. 145); whereby children are very much left to their own devices. However, they do not suggest parental failures grow out of a subcultural moral character (the problem family), but are a reflection of the poverty syndrome. They see the failure of the family to act in a protective capacity, in situational terms, i.e. arising from lack of material resources and strong feelings of powerlessness.

Wilson and Herbert consider that environmental factors outweigh heredity in terms of explaining the behaviour and abilities of their sample children. They are clear about what they call co-

variance, the relationship between brightness and rearing patterns, whereby the latter restrict a child's opportunity to exploit
his/her full potential. They conclude their book with the practical
and moral challenge: 'In the final analysis the problem of
disadvantaged children does not lie in genetic or in psychological deficits, it lies in an unequal distribution of the resources of
our society. The position of the children who grow up in poverty
is one of hope, because their disadvantage given the will can be
eliminated' (p. 198).

Children in Adversity (Wedge and Essen, 1982) asks similar
questions to Wilson and Herbert about the benefits of education,
although methodologically they are not parallel. The work is of
particular interest looking at children on the brink of adulthood.
The vast majority of the disadvantaged expected to leave school
at 16, often mentioning that their family needed the money, so it
was not just a question of poor motivation. Attainment was
lower, those disadvantaged at either 11 or 16 being seven times
more likely to be unable to do basic calculations and ten times as
likely not to be able to read well enough for everyday needs. The
disadvantaged were ten times more likely to be ascertained
educationally sub-normal. Those who had been disadvantaged at
11 but not at 16 (see Table 5.1, p. 74) were still suffering from
this poor relative position they had when starting secondary
school. Poor progress was not related to low initial ability as
more able children in the disadvantaged group seemed to be held
back in a similar way. 'It seems to be the disadvantaged status
itself which is associated with the poor progress' (p. 73). As far as
behaviour at school and adjustment at home were concerned, it
was clear that disadvantaged children, according to the reports
of their parents and teachers, were behaving less acceptably. The
disadvantaged provide society with a group of people whose
behaviour can be seen as needing correction.

THE CYCLE OF DEPRIVATION

The causes of child maladjustment leading inevitably to the
existence of maladjusted adults and parents is obviously a crucial
issue in political terms, *vis-à-vis* the costs to the welfare state. Sir
Keith Joseph in the early 1970s posited the concept of the 'cycle
of deprivation' which spawned much literature and debate. The
original focus of the cycle of deprivation thesis was experiences

of parenting during childhood would effect styles of parenting a generation later.

Families at Risk (Madge, 1983), which summarized much of the research done in this area, suggests that this continuity is clearer in the most severely deprived forms of child-rearing than in parenting in general. Poor parenting was five times as likely if parents themselves were reared in institutions provided for children in care of the state, yet a quarter of those brought up in residential care could provide good parenting, especially if they achieved a supportive marriage partnership.

Families at Risk identifies five areas which affect child rearing/deprivation:

1. The age and maturity of parents
Single-parent families, or families where there is a marriage breakdown, suffer material disadvantage and the cost to children is high. Marriages contracted at a younger age breakdown more easily, and inevitably children conceived by younger parents will be born into families that command less income. Babies born to young single parents are especially vulnerable to financial and emotional pressures and they are, it is suggested, often a status symbol of adulthood and source of attention for young women who themselves have not experienced a very satisfactory childhood.

2. The burdens carried by a family
Families with multiple problems, large numbers of children and many stresses upon them will find attentive child-rearing more difficult as our brief review of Wilson and Herbert's (1978) book already suggests.

3. Consistency and change in the lives of children
Disruption led on from one generation to another. Changes in parents, housing and family composition all took their toll.

4. The dynamics and support within the family
If the parents had a stable marriage and there was good quality interraction with and between parents, children benefited. (Brown and Harris's (1978) classic work on the social causes of depression points to an increased chance of depression among mothers lacking an intimate confiding relationship. Outside relationships with friends or peers are important for single

parents as is the existence of a supporting relationship with their own mother.)

5. The effect of particular experiences and characteristics
Inevitably and reassuringly, individual differences explain different responses to stress and problems. One cannot predict exactly if or when mental ill-health will affect parents, and children themselves have different capabilities and levels of resilience.

Madge (1983) argues that children have four main areas of need:

1. Physical care.
2. Emotional support which must be reliable and consistent.
3. Social interaction.
4. Intellectual stimulation.

These needs are not of course separate but each one feeds the other. She agrees with other authors we have already mentioned in saying

> physical growth and well-being, behaviour and progress at school are the main areas in which family neglect is likely to be reflected ... nevertheless behavioural expressions cannot be neatly related to specific problems as not all children relate to adversity in the same way (p. 7).

Some act out, some are withdrawn and anxious and depressed.

> The significance of signs of unusual behaviour should be judged principally by their intensity, the length of time they last, their rarity among children of a similar age and the presence of suffering on the part of the child. Strong concern should be felt for children with particularly persistent problems, especially when there is some suggestion that difficulty in one context is leading to problems in another (p. 7).

Yet for all this individual psychological approach, Madge acknowledges a broadly based aetiology for child behaviour problems and concludes, 'It is quite apparent that the causes of family difficulties are just as likely to originate within society or the community as within the family itself and accordingly action needs to be taken on several fronts' (p. 215).

PUBLIC ISSUES BEFORE PERSONAL TROUBLES

As is by now clear, the general approach adopted in this chapter is to consider psychological factors within the context of a sociological approach. Such an approach is radical in that it sees economic and social circumstances as the boundaries within which individual beliefs, attitudes and achievements may occur. Moral character does not predate and formulate life chances; rather, as Holman (1978) quoted earlier in this chapter suggests, personal adaptation occurs within the constraints of existing social structure. The relationship of personal troubles to public issues is regarded by many as the central issue in social science. Durkheim's classic study on 'Suicide', although now accepted as having methodological problems, is nevertheless seen as demonstrating the relationship between suicide and institutional features of society as a whole: marriage, family life, widowhood and religion. Although cause and effect is always complex and arguable in this field, in Durkheim's study it was possible to move from correlations (that depression is more common among women who are widowed) to statements about causality (that widowhood can bring about depression). An article by Clark (1987) spells out how modern-day divorce rates are four times higher in Social Class V than among professional groups, and the rates are highest of all among the unemployed. The causes and correlations are not impossible to guess.

Brown and Harris's (1978) work, already mentioned, on the social origins of depression, provides findings which can help us move from the wider scope of the first half of the chapter to consider how the caring professions in the inner city might approach their work. Brown and Harris are clear that psychiatric disorder is common among working-class women in London, but not in a rural population in Scotland. They studied 220 women in 1969/71 and 238 in 1974/5 in Camberwell and 154 in North Uist in the Outer Hebrides in 1975.

The women studied in Camberwell were only at high risk of developing depression when they had children at home. There were definite links with social class. Working-class women with children at home were four times more likely to suffer from a definite psychiatric disorder compared to their middle-class peers. The study distinguishes:

1. Provoking agents which influence when the depression occurs: i.e.

loss or threat of loss;
long term difficulty;

2. vulnerability factors which influences whether the provoking agents have any effect: i.e.

lack of intimate tie with, particularly but not exclusively, boyfriend/husband;
loss of mother, not father, before the age of eleven;
three or more children under fourteen at home; and

3. Symptom formation factors which influence the severity and form of the depressive disorder: i.e.

severe event occurring after onset of marginal depressive state;
past loss of immediate family in childhood or adolescence.

Using this model, Brown and Harris build up a picture of working-class women experiencing more severe life events and major difficulties (housing, finance, husband, child) which reflect inner city stresses. However, their particular point is that vulnerability factors influence whether the events or difficulties (provoking agents) actually bring about depression, which might have been resisted by somebody who was less vulnerable. They do suggest, housing is particularly influential on the onset of psychiatric disorder.

Levels of psychiatric disorder in the Camberwell study are very high, with 15% suffering a definitive affective disorder in the three months prior to interview. Half of these disorders seem to have begun in the previous year and a half were chronic, i.e. more or less continuous for more than a year. The researchers thought all the 15% had shown symptoms which were severe enough to warrant treatment. The survey suggested an additional 18% of women were suffering from a borderline condition. Paradoxically, in some cases very depressed women with children suggested that it was only the responsibility of the children that stopped them harming themselves, and the survey established that women with three or more children at home, although as depressed as other women, were less likely to have consulted a general practitioner about their depression. For agencies drawing conclusions from their referrals, or busy doctors believing that an empty surgery means a healthy practice, such research is sobering.

Brown and Harris reflect on the relationship between situations and perceptions of situations by those who are depressed. This is obviously a vital question when building a causal model. They ask, 'Just how much, for instance, of the difficulty of women with young children stems from the circumstances of their task and how much from a sense of doing work that is undervalued in a society geared to reward through employment' (p. 290). They are also aware of the opportunities middle-class women may have 'because of the greater variety of their lives and a greater input of positive experiences, which enable them to hope for better things more positively. . . . Adjustment in adversity may prove to be largely a matter of how to sustain hope for better things' (p. 291).

The implications of this approach are multifactorial explanations of depression breaking down traditional divisions between the various parts of the welfare state and the methods employed. 'Once it can be accepted that in many cases a combination of chemotherapy and psychotherapy needs supplementing with social changes, such as work or regular meaningful activity outside the home, the role of medical and social agencies in the treatment of depression should merge into a new perspective' (p. 291). This eclectic approach to helping seems to recommend itself because it may be considerably more effective than isolated professionalism. It exposes all helping agencies to the challenge of social science and the need to understand their professional practice within a much broader context.

HEALTH FOR ALL

The health service is probably the welfare expenditure that receives most universal support – everyone uses it at times. The principle of free service at point of demand is somewhat breached with dental and ophthalmic charges, but the nation might at least be proud of the free health care provided for its children. Yet, research has documented over and over again that social class and place of residence do influence health.

Although the infant mortality rate has continued to fall this century, the gap between the Registrar General's five social group categories (group III is split into manual and non-manual) continues and in some cases is widened. This of course is not solely a British phenomenon.

Table 5.1   Total Infant Mortality (0–11 months) 1970–2 per 1000 Live and Still Births

Social Group	I	II	IIIN	IIIM	IV	V	All infants
Males	13.60	15.21	16.91	19.06	22.03	34.73	19.91
Females	9.61	11.94	11.99	14.79	16.95	26.67	15.27

OPCS (1985).

Accidents which cause 30% of child deaths show the sharpest class gradient, with other causes such as pneumonia and bronchitis following suit, although the contrast here between the classes is not quite so severe. Wilson and Herbert's (1978) identification of the lower levels of supervision or 'chaperonage' poorer parents can give, become very relevant when considering boys in group V have a much greater chance of dying of fire, falls or drowning than those in group I, and the ratio for traffic accidents is 7 to 1.

Infant mortality rates are also significant when considering country of birth of mother, with mothers born in Pakistan suffering a 22 per 1000 rate in 1977 compared with 13 per thousand of mothers born in the United Kingdom. The rate also falls as one moves from the north to the south of England and is lower in rural than urban areas. The differing rates up and down the country reflect the distribution of 'disadvantaged' children that was revealed when we looked at the findings of the National Child Development Study. Furthermore, the fall in mortality rate from north to south is still detectable even allowing for socio-economic inequalities. The Health Service is making attempts to deal with this unequal service provision by redistribution of resources (the RAWP system).

Blaxter (1981), in reviewing the health disadvantages of children, says:

> Poverty, poor housing, vulnerable family structures and disturbed family relationships, pollution and the environment of urban deprivation, lack of knowledge and inability to make the most efficient use of what the health services have to offer, are all indicted ... a great deal of effort has gone into the task of proving again and again that these socially associated differences in the health status of children do exist: almost as if this were something that society did not wish to believe and had to rediscover at regular intervals (p. 219).

For our purposes, the Black Report on *Inequalities in Health* (DHSS, 1980). is central to the question of family and child health. It recommended that health and social services should adopt a three-fold scheme of priorities:

1. Priority for children to have a better start in life.
2. Priority for disabled people to improve the quality of their life and avoid institutional care.
3. Priority for preventive and educational action to encourage good health.

Its conclusions are not primarily concerned with curative medicine *per se* (although its members were split as to whether money should be moved from curative to preventive work), but rather look at broader measures which will combat the disadvantages in health that the poor experience. For example, the report recommended special health and social development experimental programmes in a selected number of areas — Salford, Thamesside, Gateshead, Liverpool, South Tyneside, Tower Hamlets, Durham, Bolton, Wirral and North Tyneside — which in descending order have the highest death rates standardized per population and age/sex distribution. The report as an example supporting its desire for initiatives in these special areas, mentions Gateshead (third on the infant mortality list for the country). Gateshead has in some of its local wards an infant mortality rate three times as high as in other wards and the wards with the highest infant mortality rates were also wards with the smallest proportions of population in social groups I and II.

The Black Report recommends various preventive strategic and organizational changes based on the 'acknowledgement of the multi-causal nature of health inequalities, within which inequalities in the material conditions of living loom large' (p. 207). The Report sees childhood as the 'period of life at which intervention could most hopefully weaken the continuing association between health and class' (p. 207). Its recommendations include:

1. School health statistics measuring hearing, height, etc., in relation to the occupational class of families.

2. Improving information and preventive programmes in relation to child accidents.

3. Improving the nutritional surveillance level of the National Food Survey.

4. Improving measurement of real incomes.

5. Inequalities in health should be a DHSS research priority.

6. Health resources should be allocated according to need and shifted towards community care, including ante-natal, post-natal and child health services.

7. The general practitioner service, which can be inadequate and single-handed in inner city areas, should be related to standardized mortality ratios and should be backed up in areas where shortfall is discovered by above-average numbers of community nurses.

8. Accessibility to, and facilities at, ante-natal and child health services should be reviewed.

9. Local authorities should improve their day care for under-fives and the role of day nurseries and nursery schools should be reviewed so that both meet the needs of children for education and care.

10. School health care should be revitalized and better linked with general practice. Follow-up in areas of special need and for certain types of families should be improved.

11. The abolition of child proverty should be adopted as a national goal for the 1980s. Higher child benefits with increased rates to cover the extra costs of older children, increased maternity grant and an infant care allowance were also recommended.

12. School meals should be provided as a right.

These proposals would cost a lot of money, £2 billion according to the then (1980) Secretary of State, Patrick Jenkin, who gave the proposals a very lukewarm response. It is not this chapter's job to discuss the cost of the welfare state, but at present we are not out of step with our neighbours in terms of health care expenditure as a percentage of GNP, but implementing the Black Report would mean a clear and new political priority being agreed.

The argument for it is the rights of children to get a more equal start in life. The argument against it is other more important political priorities, and the electorate's ambivalence about increased rates of tax. At the time of writing, funding the National Health Service and alternative ways of so doing are high on the political agenda.

THE RACIAL DIMENSION

In 1985 there were 2.4 million non-whites in the country and it is important to remember two-fifths of the non-white population were born in the U.K. Since the last war, black people from ex-British colonies have settled in the inner city, forced to congregate, as poor people must, in run-down areas. Only recently has there been a net inflow of people coming into Britain (returning Britons and Common Market workers have tipped the balance). The broader picture is of the indigenous white population moving to richer expanding economic areas as black people from the Asian sub-continent and the Caribbean came to Britain.

Although we now have recently had over 3 million unemployed, it is important to remember that this country actively recruited people in places like Barbados for lowly paid jobs in transport and catering. Similarly, northern European countries sucked in Turks, Moroccans and Algerians to fuel their expanding economies.

The 1948 Nationality Act opened the way for immigration. Subsequently, the Government has sought both to legislate to improve race relations while also feeling the need to limit the number of black people entering the country. Thus the experience for black people is somewhat contradictory as the control process discriminates in favour of those who have U.K. roots and therefore against the black new Commonwealth citizens, while the thrust of the anti-discrimination legislation that has been passed is egalitarian.

There is no doubt that race and law and order have become intertwined in the media and therefore in the consciousness of each one of us. There is also no doubt that black people can, and do, feel severely discomforted by the response of the majority community. They experience discrimination in the areas of housing, education and employment. Lord Scarman's report to the Government on the Brixton Riots of 1981 acknowledges this discrimination quite clearly and also poses the problem of how to police the inner cities sensitively.

It is important to remember that the majority of black people in this country are able to live decent lives, but also it is the case they often feel less identified with the main stream of the society. There is much discussion as to whether special help needs to be provided or whether they must just get along as best as they can ('When in Rome ...'). Urban aid and other forms of help are provided to the inner cities with racial harmony an important motivational factor shared across the political spectrum. There is much academic and political debate about whether the money is spent to help people in the inner cities or just to contain them: i.e., for whose benefit is urban aid really spent? There is also much debate about what sort of projects are most effective in terms of benefiting inner cities.

Scarman's report (1981) recommends reviewing housing policies, with special reference to involving the community, rehabilitation of existing property and a review of local authority tenancy allocations. He recommends a government initiative in ethnic minority education, pointing to provision for under-fives, special training for teachers in relation to minority needs and expectations, the teaching of English and the involvement of parents in schools. Scarman in his conclusions says that unemployment weighs 'disproportionately heavily on black people. . . . There can be no doubt that unemployment is a major factor in the complex pattern of conditions which lies at the root of the disorders in Brixton and elsewhere' (para. 8.48).

Racial prejudice is most hateful when its destructive effect can be seen in the eyes and hearts of black children. *Faith in the City* talks of children's abilities being stereotyped in terms of sport or dance. Under-achievement is not confined to those of West Indian origin. When the Archbishop's commission visited Bradford there was considerable concern from the Asian community (pp. 302–3).

It is important to realize that the subconscious views of the superiority of whiteness that we should all be struggling to overcome are based on a long history. It is important for black and white to appreciate some of the history of slavery and imperial domination that still haunts our inner city life. We all need to support strong black identities that are positive and stand in their own right. There is a tradition of colour blindness which in fact denies the important meaning of being a black person. Black is different, equal and good.

Halsey (1981) quotes from a 1974 Central Policy Review Staff Report, presented to the Government but never published, which says:

There are uncomfortable parallels between the situation of Britain's coloured population and that of the Catholics in

Northern Ireland. For 50 years British Governments con-
doned discrimination and deprivation in Ulster, and in the
end Ulster blew up in their face. We believe that not only for
reasons of social justice but also to preserve social stability
and order in the longer term more should be done to deal
with the problems of race relations in this country (p. 63).

When trying to provide sensitive and appropriate services for
black people, it is important to make sure that the professional
staff delivering those services reflect the racial mix of the
community which they serve, and are encouraged by that service
to make sure its help is appropriate for and accepted by ethnic
minorities. Because of the disadvantages already structured into
our society this demands training initiatives to make sure that
suitably qualified black people are available to present themselves at all levels in the welfare state. Issues about language and
translation services, especially in relation to Asian mothers and
their families, need addressing. How do you work if you cannot
understand what people say? It is also vital that all professional
workers give real credibility to the views articulated by black
people, even if their initial reaction may see those views as
extreme. As black people's experience is so different, it may be
hard to 'hear' what they are saying. However, so to do is a key
element in real professionalism.

BEING PROFESSIONAL IN THE INNER CITY

Having considered the explanations of poverty, deprivation and
even depression, and adopted a stance that says they are not
intrinsic to particular families or individuals, but can be
accounted for, in part at least, by socio-economic processes, the
question arises, is this knowledge really useful and can it
therefore be a springboard to action?

Brown and Harris (1978) suggest traditional case work or
social workers may not help depressed women, and Wilson and
Herbert (1978), looking at their sample, found it hard to
distinguish between families allocated social workers and those
who are not. All the professional groups have areas of unease
where they go through the motions but are dubious about the
outcome.

If many of the constraints on professionals helping children
and families in the inner cities may be to do with factors outside

the orbit of their disciplines this may seem depressing, but it does require of health workers, from consultant to cleaner, as a minimum:

1. That they are aware of the external constraints that mould people's lives and do not assume they have experienced life as their patients/clients have. Readers may find themselves working across gaps of class, race and income. To bridge this gap it requires an assessment of how the person/patient/client sees themself and the helping services. Start where the individual is and do not assume he/she will be understanding or appreciative of the service. Women know how patronizing men can be. Professional women can replicate this in their work with disadvantaged groups, if they do not make an effort to 'put themselves in the other person's shoes'.

2. That they do not practise in a way that denies the structural problems of their patients/clients. When the temptation is great to make moral judgements, i.e. lazy, manipulative, dirty, then is the time to step back and look at the wider context of the person's life. Where has their economic, educational and social opportunities set them in life? What family history do they have and how do those patterns influence them today and reflect in the way they bring up their own children?*

3. That they positively acquire skills which complement this eclectic structural explanatory framework. This may imply learning about and involvement with preventive, educative and self-help programmes. It is important to help people link the personal and the public parts of their lives. Helping isolated people to get involved in group or self-help activities can be very time consuming, yet the discovery that other people have problems, but also have some fight in them, is powerful help. The caveat is that just referring individuals to the playgroup or the community centre is not enough, it has got to be checked out to see it matches the needs of the individual and is not as judgemental and rejecting as other experiences may have been. Ideally, facilities are organized around the needs of identified groups of people, so matching individuals or families to the right supportive resource is important.

*Those with children know how all parents find themselves dealing with their own children in the same way they were dealt with as children, even if intellectually they know it may not be the best way. Also children become other people as well as themselves in generational history, i.e. just like her mother or just like Uncle Bob.

All this may sound hopelessly idealistic and yet there are examples of programmes constructed in line with this kind of thinking.

In West London on a large ex-GLC estate there is a mental health project which seeks to combine a four-tier approach to women vulnerable to depression. The aim is to move women through a process of psychotherapy, groupwork, mental health education to the eventual stimulation of mutual help initiatives within the neighbourhood. In stage one the question is 'What does your depression mean and where does it come from?' moving on to, in a group setting, 'What do you want of yourself and others?' and finally 'How can we change the world we inhabit?' The founder of this project, Sue Holland, quotes as an example of what they are trying to achieve, an Afro-Caribbean Group which brought together black women who had known severe depression and were working on relating their suffering to the wider context of their collective history and present life in Britain. Sue Holland's project has spawned its own self-help group called Women's Action for Mental Health (WAMH), which constitutes the end of the process from psychotherapy to community action. It provides a good example of how the concept of changing private troubles into public issues can be turned into real services dealing with health.

Community resources to link people into are there – racial and religious groups, self-help groups or local pressure groups. Where is your local Pre-School Playgroup's organizer? Do MIND or Mencap have a local branch? Can your local Campaign for Racial Equality help? Is there a Victims of Crime Support Scheme locally? What is available at the health centre nearest to where someone lives? The Town Hall will have local information and there is likely to be a coordinator for local voluntary groups. Social Services, either in the social work department of the hospital or in the area team, could give you some useful addresses. Hospitals are a focus for charitable and voluntary help. Get to know the area you work in and the resources that are available to support the good health of the individuals in the community.

The policy recommendations arising from the Black Report (DHSS, 1980), see p. 83, may again seem distant from the individual professional, but awareness of where the needs are likely to be greatest and the take-up poor is a step that each individual can take. Equally important is organizing personal

priorities so that need rather than demand is the first consideration. Also, when opportunities arise, individuals can provide a
commentary back into the NHS about the problems that are
encountered and the constraints to good health that are experienced in the inner cities. Awareness that high technology
medicine, important though it is, will never solve the health
problems the Black Report spells out, provides a backdrop
against which health care in the inner cities can be practised.

Underlying all of what is said in this last section is the
importance of making constructive listening relationships.
Wendy Savage's (1986) book on her difficult experiences as a
gynaecologist in Hackney suggests a way a consultant can
realign her relationships with her patients (controversial though
this may be to some). It is suggested by Wendy Savage (1986)
that the principle of engaging the patient and giving her view
credence, time-consuming though it may be, will in the end
provide the best sort of health care.

It is important to acknowledge how different the experience of
working out in the community visiting can be in comparison to
working in a hospital or other care institution. However, the
comments here and the conclusions drawn are equally relevant to
the hospital setting perhaps even more important in a way. The
patient in bed is inevitably less able to present the world he/she
comes from and the way he/she thinks, not only because he/she
is ill but because of the powerlessness even the highly articulate
feel in the hospital system.

CONCLUSIONS

This chapter, in the material and ideas it has presented, runs the
risk of seeming strategically orientated and therefore distant to
the individual health worker. Job descriptions do not include the
demands made on professionals in this chapter, and the time is
just not available, some would say, to work in the ways
suggested, even if there is no personal animosity to such an
approach. This criticism is acknowledged. It has been taken into
consideration in the writing. Nevertheless, it is suggested that
each of us can be aware on a day-to-day basis that

  1. Healthy people need material resources, a social context
     and community support.

2. Good practice requires listening professional relationships.
3. The language of medicine may not only need translating into other languages but also into everyday English.
4. Class based inequalities in health are an important issue and undermine the effectiveness of individuals practising in the inner cities. Racism within individuals and society can be a further block to minorities getting a good service. Everyone needs to examine very carefully their own views about race.
5. If the health service is based on the principle of equality, as it is, then professionals involved, individually and collectively, have a duty to see that every family and every child they come into contact with gets care based on need and provided within an appreciation of the social and economic constraints that prevail in that family.

Table 5.2   Current Income Support Rates as from April 1988

Couple −	
Both under 18	£38.80
One or both over 18	£51.45
Lone parent −	
Under 18	£19.40
18 or over	£33.40
Dependent children −	
Under 11	£10.75
11–15	£16.10
16–17	£19.40
18	£26.05
Additional premiums −	
Family premium	£6.15
Disabled child premium	£6.15
Lone-parent premium	£3.70

Example:
One parent family with two children under 11 −

Lone parent	£33.40	
Two children	£21.50	
Lone-parent premium	£3.70	
Family premium	£6.15	
	Total	£64.75

(20% of the rates must be paid out of this weekly allowance.)

REFERENCES

Abel-Smith B. and Townsend P. (1965). *The Poor and the Poorest.* London: G. Bell.

Archbishop of Canterbury's Commission on Urban Priority Areas (1985). *Faith in the City* (Chairman: Sir Richard O'Brien). London: Church Publishing.

Blaxter M. (1981). *The Health of Children: A Review of the Place of Health in Cycles of Disadvantage.* London: Heinemann Educational.

Briggs A. (1961). *Seebohm Rountree.* London: Longmans.

Brown G. W. and Harris T. (1978) *The Social Origins of Depression.* London: Tavistock.

Clark D. (1987). The family in crisis. New Society Series 2. 'Wedlocked Britain'. *New Society* **13,** Mar. 12–15.

Conway J. and Kemp P. (1985). *Bed and Breakfast: Slum Housing of the Eighties.* London: SHAC.

Department of Environment (1977). *A Policy for the Inner Cities.* Cmnd 6845. London: HMSO.

Department of Health and Social Security (1980). *Inequalities in Health.* Report of a research working group (Chairman: Sir Douglas Black). London: HMSO.

Essen J. and Wedge P. (1982). *Continuities in Childhood Disadvantage.* London: Heinemann Educational.

The Guardian (1985). Editorial, 3 Dec.

Halsey A. H. (1981) *Change in British Society.* 2nd edn. Oxford: Oxford University Press.

Harrison P. (1985). *Inside the Inner City: Life Under the Cutting Edge.* Revsd. edn. Harmondsworth: Penguin.

Hirsch F. (1976). *The Social Limits of Growth.* Boston, Mass: Harvard University Press.

Holman R. (1978). *Poverty Explanations of Social Deprivation.* London: Robertson.

Jordan B. (1981). *Automatic Poverty.* London: Routledge & Kegan Paul.

Le Grand J. (1982). *The Strategy of Equality.* London: George Allen & Unwin.

Mack J. and Lansley S. (1985). *Poor Britain.* London: George Allen & Unwin.

Madge N. (ed.) (1983). *Families at risk.* London: Heinemann Educational.

OPCS (1985). *Mortality Statistics 1984.* London: HMSO.

Piachaud D. (1979). *The Cost of a Child.* London: Child Poverty Action Group.

Prince Philip (1986). *Inquiry into British Housing.* Chairman: HRH Duke of Edinburgh. London: National Federation of Housing Associations.

Savage W. (1986). *A Savage Inquiry: Who controls childbirth?* London: Virago Press.

Scarman (Lord) (1981). *The Brixton Disorders 10–12 April 1981*: Report of an Enquiry. Cmnd 8427. London: HMSO.

Wedge P. and Essen J. (1982). *Children in Adversity*. London: Pan.

Wedge P. and Prosser H. (1973). *Born to Fail?* London: Arrow Books.

Wilson H. and Herbert G. W. (1978). *Parents and Children in the Inner City*. London: Routlege & Kegan Paul.

USEFUL ADDRESS

Women's Action for Mental Health
c/o 131 Bloemfontein Road, London W12.

6

General Practice

BRIAN JARMAN

THE DEVELOPMENT AND CHARACTERISTICS OF GENERAL PRACTICE

To appreciate the situation of general practitioners in inner cities at the end of the twentieth century it is helpful first to consider the development of the system of general practice which we have in the United Kingdom. General practitioners were the successors of the apothecaries who had first emerged as a body in the seventeeth century. In the nineteenth century general practitioners were paid by friendly societies and working men's clubs to certify periods of sickness so that workers could receive compensation when they were off work due to illness. The workers were paid from a fund to which they contributed by means of weekly payments. In addition to certifying periods of sickness, the general practitioners also provided general medical services and dispensed medicines. They received between two and four shillings for each person in the club per year for providing these services. This was the beginning of the capitation system of payment of general practitioners which has persisted to the present day, although now in a considerably modified form.

The friendly societies and working-men's clubs had a considerable degree of control over the doctors who worked for them. If they were dissatisfied with the general practitioners' services they could be dismissed with little right of appeal. The capitation payments which general practitioners received were small and they depended to a significant extent on the number of private patients they could attract. General practitioners came to resent these conditions of work and the relatively low pay. In 1911, following the introduction of social security legislation in Germany at the end of the nineteenth century, Lloyd George introduced the National Health Insurance (NHI) Act. General practitioners were pleased to cooperate because the terms of service represented an improvement in their conditions of work. Under the Act wage earners in a family paid four pence per week and the Government five pence per week to cover sickness, disability and maternity benefits as well as general medical services for those who were insured under the scheme, without further cost at the time the service was provided. General practitioners were able to take on to their lists patients who lived near their surgeries (not just those who were members of a particular club or friendly society) and they were given a considerable say in the local administration of their services. In addition they were able to choose whether or not to accept patients on to their list (just as patients were free to change doctors if they wished).

Between 1911 and 1948 the extent of the population covered by the NHI Act increased from about one-third to about two-thirds because other groups such as the unemployed were brought in. However, a significant proportion of women were still not covered and hospital services were also not provided under the scheme – the poor depending mainly on the voluntary hospitals which gave free care. There was a move in 1920 to form health centres with salaried general practitioners, community nursing services, social facilities and even a few beds, all under the control of the local authorities, as the result of a report of a committee chaired by Lord Dawson. This was not popular with most general practitioners as they feared a salaried service and local authority control. Health centres did not develop in any significant way until the Family Doctors' Charter of 1966. In 1948, with the introduction of the National Health Service, general practitioners accepted an extension of the Lloyd George panel system to cover the whole population. They had initially opposed the idea of universal coverage in the hope that a proportion of the richer section of society would still continue to pay their general practitioners privately. However, they eventually agreed to full coverage of the population in exchange for a reassurance that the conditions which were operative under the panel system would continue more or less unchanged after 1948, with general practitioners remaining as independent contractors and having a significant influence, both locally and nationally, on the way the service was administered.

Between 1948 and 1966 was a period of relative decline in general practitioner services at the time when hospital services and scientific medicine were expanding. The payment of general practitioners almost entirely by means of capitation until 1966 meant that there was competition between doctors to attract patients on to their lists. However, there was little incentive, having registered the patients, to provide services for these patients because the annual capitation fee was fixed. In fact, the reverse was the case because the less the general practitioners did for their patients, the less costly it was for them in terms of time and money. Although this had the advantage that there was no incentive to provide unnecessary services (as might occur if payment was on an item of service basis), it was also not 'cost-effective' to take on 'difficult' patients who might provide a lot of work for the same fixed annual fee. These considerations are still relevant today, particularly in inner city areas, as is shown below.

General practitioners were generally dissatisfied with these arrangements for payment purely by means of capitation and the type of service that this system tended to promote. In 1965 they put considerable pressure on the Government (by threatening to resign from the NHS) to introduce the Family Doctor's Charter of 1966. This changed the method of payment of general practitioners from capitation to one where only half their income was received by this means and a form of salary was introduced (known as a basic practice allowance) which made up about a quarter of their income. Payments were introduced for practising in group practice and for providing proven preventive services, such as immunizations and cervical smears, and these roughly made up the remaining quarter of their income. In addition, the cost of the rent and rates of approved premises and 70% of the cost of members of certain categories of ancillary staff were reimbursed to the general practitioners, together with the cost of employing a trainee in a training practice. These were incentives for providing a better service rather than giving the general practitioner a higher income. From this time onwards the standards of general practitioners and their general morale have increased, primary health care teams have developed and there has been a considerable increase in the number of general practitioners practising in health centres. General practice is by far the most popular choice of medical students, about half of whom give it as their career preference. In 1981 three years of postgraduate vocational training became compulsory for doctors wishing to enter general practice – this comprises two years in approved hospital specialties and one year in an approved, and regularly inspected, training practice.

The improvements in general practice which resulted after the 1966 Family Doctors' Charter were substantial. Even though general practitioners have remained as self-employed independent contractors as they were before 1948 (rather than salaried employees as are all other doctors in the NHS), there are several advantages of the system which has evolved. There is virtually complete coverage of the whole country with a personal doctor (99% of the population, although less in inner city areas) providing continuing care to families, each patient being registerd with their general practitioner for an average of about ten years. For many elderly and disabled people have frequent contacts with their general practitioners.

Table 6.1 Use of Some Health and Social Services by Elderly People Aged 65 or over in the Month before Interview

	% all elderly
Doctor in surgery	24
Doctor at home	11
Doctor at surgery or home	33
District nurse/health visitor	8
Chiropodist	9
Home help	10
Meals-on-wheels	3
Lunch out (lunch club/day centre)	4
Day centre	5

Source: General Household Survey, 1986.
100% base sample = 3760.
Question asked: 'Which of these services did you make use of last month?'

Almost all general practice is provided under the auspices of the NHS rather than privately. This is in spite of the fact that general practitioners are able to accept as many private patients as they wish (as non-NHS patients), but cannot treat their NHS patients privately. The General Household Survey shows that only about 1% of consultations in the community are with private general practitioners. The costs of general practitioner services represent only 7% of the cost of the NHS. This excludes the costs of the drugs they prescribe, the investigations done at their request in hospital and the cost of other members of the primary care team provided by the District Health Authority, Local Authorities or voluntary bodies. About 80% of episodes of illness are covered within the primary care setting without any treatment in hospital: hospitals account for about 62% of NHS costs. General practice has proved to be flexible; for example in adapting to situations such as rural areas, where there are special payments for rural practice, and to cover the highlands and islands of Scotland.

The Medical Practice Committee was formed in 1948 to ensure an even distribution of doctors. Areas where the average list size of general practitioners is high (designated areas) have incentives to encourage general practitioners to practise in those areas. Where the average list size of general practitioners is low (restricted areas) no new doctors are allowed to practise under the auspices of the NHS. This results in a very even distribution of general practitioners in the United Kingdom. This is probably the most even distribution of primary care doctors of any country in the world – the average list size being about 2000 patients per doctor with nearly two-thirds of list sizes being within the range of 1900 to 2100 (in 1988).

The main problems in general practice which have not yet been fully dealt with are:

1. Quality assessment and assurance;
2. Comprehensive measures to promote health; and
3. The problems of inner cities.

The Government's 1987 White Paper on Primary Health Care, which is discussed below, has attempted to tackle all of these deficiencies.

INNER CITIES

The difficulties for inner cities arise from three main facts:

1. There is a higher concentration of *patients* with characteristics which are thought to increase the workload or pressure on the services of primary care workers.

2. There are additional difficulties, because of the inner city environment, related to the *working conditions* for primary care workers in these areas.

3. There is, as yet, little or *no adaptation of the services to the conditions in inner cities.*

Surveys have shown that in inner cities there are high concentrations of *patients* who tend to produce greater pressure on the services of primary care workers wherever they practice. These include such groups as elderly people living alone, one-parent families, the homeless, ethnic minorities and also the unemployed and working-class sections of the population and those with higher mobility. There are also higher levels of morbidity and mortality in inner city areas.

In addition to having, in general, a more difficult group of patients, in urban areas there are also factors which make it more difficult to provide good *services* in these very areas where patients have higher needs. The cost of building and the problem of finding and developing sites in inner city areas make it difficult to establish adequate premises for primary health care teams and there is no variation to allow for this in the cost rent scheme by which general practitioners are able to build their own premises, nor is there any special allowance for health authorities to provide health centres in deprived areas. The cost of living and working in inner cities are high (particularly in the West End of London), but again there is no allowance for this in the expenses element of the payment to general practitioners. General practitioners are the only group of workers in the NHS in London who do not receive a London Allowance. A further difficulty arises from the fact that in areas where general practitioners are keeping relatively low list sizes (either to enable them to deal more effectively with the greater workload or because there may be less stress and a higher income from non-NHS work) the area average list size is inevitably lower than the national average. This means that under the rules of the Medical Practices Committee no new general practitioners are allowed to practise in these areas. Young trainees who come from the Inner City Medical Schools cannot get into general practice in their locality. The average age of the general practitioners increases and, if list sizes are being kept low, patients find difficulty getting on to general practitioners' lists.

As a consequence of the operation of the mechanisms described above, the factors characterizing general practice in many inner city areas, and in Inner London particularly, are a predominance of elderly single-handed general practitioners and poor standards of practice premises. There is some doubt expressed by nursing managers regarding the appropriateness of nursing attachments to general practices in inner city areas, partly because of the lack of group practices and partly because of the lack of adequate general practitioner premises for the nurses to work from. The percentage of community nurses attached to general practices in inner city areas to form primary care teams is therefore low.

A survey by Hughes and Roberts (1980) showed that in Inner London community nurses tend to be younger and stay less time in post than in the outer areas (nearly half leaving annually in some districts). The average number of nurses per head of the population is a little higher than outside the inner city areas but the establishment is often not filled. Nurses have the problems of higher living costs in inner urban areas or expensive travelling costs to work, particularly in Inner London. Many of the inner city teaching hospitals train community nurses. This helps them with the difficult task of recruitment but, after working a year or two in the district where they trained, these nurses often can not afford, or do not want, to settle down more permanently, make their homes and bring up a family in these districts. Thus the high turnover of community nurses in inner city areas arises. For general practitioners a high turnover is, fortunately, not such a pronounced problem – not because the same conditions do not exist for them, because they do, but because general practitioners are dependent on their registered list of patients for their income and they are not easily able to change their practice area and register a new group of patients. About 5% of general practitioners leave the medical list in inner city areas annually, about a half as a result of retirement and the figures for inner cities are similar to those which apply nationally. They therefore have to adapt to inner city conditions in other ways.

Some of the ways that general practitioners have of compensating for higher living and working costs and more stressing patients are to reduce their expenditure on patient services and to be selective about taking on patients (or removing 'difficult' patients from their lists). This may then result in patients using hospital services more often than in other areas and is probably one of the factors contributing to higher hospitalization rates (standardized for age and sex) in inner city areas. Other factors also lead to higher hospitalization rates; these are high illness rates, poor housing and home care conditions and greater availability of hospital services and all of these are also operative in inner city areas. Age/sex standardized hospitalization rates in inner cities are up to 45% above national rates and bed usage rates up to 70% above the values expected based on the age and sex structures of their populations. This of course adds an additional financial strain to inner city districts which are losing resources under the Resource Allocation Working Party (RAWP) formula. The RAWP formula at present allows for differences in Standardized Mortality Ratios (SMRs) but does not take account of any of the problems related to social conditions, primary care or greater availability of hospital services.

SOLUTIONS FOR THE PROBLEMS OF PRIMARY CARE IN INNER CITIES

What is needed is some way of taking account of the variety of complex factors involved in the provision of primary health care in inner cities and making the appropriate allowances and adjustments of the service provision to compensate for the particular situations in these areas. The Acheson Report (LHPC, 1981), *Primary Health Care* in Inner London, and a report from the Royal College of General Practitioners (Jarman, 1981), as well as the Green Paper on Primary Care Services (DHSS, 1986a) and the subsequent White Paper (DHSS, 1987) have all tackled this problem. The 1979 Royal Commission on the NHS, the Harding Report on the Primary Care Team (DHSS, 1981) and the Cumberlege Report on Neighbourhood Nursing (DHSS, 1986b) have each made valuable contributions regarding the problems of inner city primary care.

The 1987 White Paper (DHSS) on improving primary health care brings together many of the topics tackled in the previous documents. It has recommended a variety of solutions to the problems and has dealt with the questions of quality control, health promotion as well as of inner cities. One of the key recommendations is of a deprived-area allowance and many of the recommendations mention special modifications of service provision in defined inner city areas. In order that these recommendations may be implemented it is essential that there is a method of identifying exactly where these areas are and that this method is agreed and accepted by those concerned.

IDENTIFYING INNER CITY AREAS

In 1981 a questionnaire was sent to one in ten general practitioners in the United Kingdom asking them to score from 0 to 9 a
series of service and social factors which they considered
increased their workload or pressure on their services when
present in their areas. From this a score was developed by taking
the values of the social variables covered in the survey from the
national census, weighting them by the general practitioners'
national average weightings and summing them to make what
was called an underprivileged area (UPA) score (Jarman, 1983
and 1984). This survey of general practitioners was repeated for
all of the community nurses in one Health Authority (Bloomsbury) and also for a sample of the health visitors in District
Health Authorities in England.

THE HEALTH VISITORS' SURVEY

A questionnaire similar to the one sent to general practitioners
was sent to a sample of Health Visitors' Association members
working as health visitors, health visitors/school nurses or as
health visitors/fieldwork teachers in English District Health
Authorities. The study was to look into factors which increase
the workload of, or contribute to the pressure on, the work of
health visitors.

In the general practitioner survey, a total of 2587 question-
naires were sent to general practitioners eligible to be included in
the survey but only 1802 (70%) were available for the analysis
because some did not reply and others did not complete the form
correctly. With the health visitor survey, approximately 900
were sent and only 663 were available for analysis (74% of the
number sent out). The questionnaire instructions were:

1. Score factors only when they are present in your health
   visiting practice.
2. Indicate 0 only when you consider the factor has no effect.
3. Indicate N/K when the effect of the factor is not known to
   you.
4. Leave the space blank if the factor is not present.

The results were broken into four main categories and the
average scores calculated for each variable in these categories.

The average scores from the health visitor survey were compared with those from the general practitioner survey and these are shown in Table 6.2 (there were some additional questions in the health visitor survey which were not sent to the general practitioners).

Considering the social factors recorded in the census, three variables – lacking amenities, ethnic groups and overcrowding of households – had similar scores in the general practitioner and health visitor surveys. The health visitor scores were higher for under-fives, unemployment, single-parent families, unskilled workers, moved house in the last year and non-married couple families. The general practitioner scores were higher for the over-65s and elderly alone (as were the scores of community nurses in the district surveyed). These differences may well indicate that the health visitors spent more of their time dealing with the groups of patients to whom they gave higher scores. Overall the differences between the health visitor and general practitioner scores were not great.

The census social variables are used to calculate the UPA scores of the populations living in geographical areas thoughout England and Wales. Only the first eight of the census social factors listed in Table 6.2 were used in the calculation and the remaining three were not used for a variety of reasons. For instance, the proportion of households lacking basic amenities was not included as it was considered that this variable no longer gives a good indication of poor housing conditions, particularly on housing estates, as they are now built to conform to standards which include basic amenities and yet are often in poor condition because of vandalism and so on. The only housing variable included was overcrowding of households.

The UPA score was constructed based on the level of each variable in each area weighted according to the weighting from the national general practitioner survey. A health visitor score was also calculated using the weightings from the health visitor survey. Before weighting, the variables were normalized (with an ARCSIN (square root of the variable) transformation to make the distributions more normal) and then standardized (by subtracting the mean and dividing by the standard deviation of the normalized values of all the areas being considered throughout the country). The sum of the weighted, standardized, normalized values of the variables for an area gave the HV score. Because the values are standardized, the average values of the UPA and HV

**Table 6.2   Comparison of Results of the Health Visitor and
General Practitioner Surveys**

The score is an estimate by health visitors or general practitioners of
the degree to which the factor concerned increases their workload or
the pressure on their services.

CENSUS SOCIAL FACTORS

Factor	Valid replies*	Mean HV score	Mean GP score
1. Elderly alone	565	4.78	6.62
2. Under fives	640	6.02	4.64
3. Single-parent families	638	5.05	3.01
4. Unskilled workers	631	4.84	2.88
5. Unemployment	629	4.92	3.34
6. Ethnic groups	573	2.27	2.50
7. Overcrowded households	605	3.18	2.88
8. Moved house in 1 year	596	3.52	2.68
9. Over-65s	578	4.59	6.19
10. Lack of amenities	601	3.43	3.60
11. Non-married couple families	620	4.23	2.71

HOUSING FACTORS

Type of housing	Valid replies*	Mean HV score
Council	626	4.20
Private	561	2.42
Temporary	516	2.39
Owner occupied	613	2.33

MISCELLANEOUS SOCIAL FACTORS

Factor	Valid replies*	Mean HV score	Mean GP score
Crime rate	556	3.01	2.30
Travel difficulties	601	3.09	3.10

SERVICE FACTORS

Factor	Valid replies*	Mean HV score	Mean GP score
HV or GP to population ratio	558	4.43	
Low expenditure on community health service	598	5.03	4.29
Low expenditure on home helps	552	4.68	4.19
Low expenditure on meals-on-wheels	527	4.21	4.19
Low expenditure on under-5 population	618	6.00	
Low expenditure on over-65 population	549	5.15	
Poor services for the elderly	556	4.88	
High proportion of single-handed GPs	502	1.70	0.93
Primary health care teams	555	3.87	2.83

*Health visitor survey.

scores for the whole country are each 0. It is found that the standard deviation of the UPA score is ± 16.7 and of the HV score is ± 20.7. The range of UPA scores for the District Health Authorities of England is from − 32.79 to + 54.89, the high scores being in the areas with the worst social conditions. For the HV score the range of values is from − 43.46 to 67.55, the greater range being related to the higher weightings given by health visitors. The correlation coefficient between the UPA and HV scores for the districts of England is 0.97 and the correlation with other indices of deprivation such as those developed by the Department of the Environment and by Professor Peter Townsend is about 0.90.

Table 6.3 gives the UPA and HV scores of the top 20 districts in England arranged in order of HV score ranking. The ranking in terms of UPA score is also given and it can be seen that there is a considerable degree of overlap between the rankings. Bloomsbury Health Authority is higher in the UPA score rank order because general practitioners give a greater weighting to the elderly alone variable and Bloomsbury has the highest proportion of elderly alone in the country. As the UPA and HV scores correlate so highly, and as the UPA score is much more generally available, it is probably adequate to use the UPA score as a measure of the potential workload or pressure on the services of health visitors as well as general practitioners. The UPA score was accepted at the 1983 general practitioner annual conference of representatives of local medical committees as a method of

Table 6.3 Ranking of DHAs of England by HV Score and UPA score
(values of each variable used for the scores are also shown.)

Department health authority name	Residential population	Elderly living alone	Children under 5 years of age	Lone parents	Unskilled	Unemployed	Overcrowded homes	Changed address	Ethnic minorities	Health visitor score	Health visitor ranking	Underprivileged area (GP) score	General practitioner ranking
Tower Hamlets	139 996	6.32	6.95	3.81	10.75	15.57	21.55	11.74	20.28	67.55	1	54.89	1
Central Manchester	115 924	5.99	6.62	4.34	9.47	20.82	16.85	11.54	16.64	65.63	2	50.83	2
City and Hackney	184 230	5.90	6.86	5.11	7.28	15.00	18.25	10.60	27.45	62.10	3	48.62	3
West Birmingham	209 907	5.07	7.29	3.38	7.83	19.70	20.43	9.21	30.14	57.11	4	44.46	5
Paddington and North Kensington	113 618	7.04	5.36	4.22	7.07	12.86	17.36	17.30	16.51	53.45	5	44.80	4

Camberwell	213 864	5.96	6.11	5.02	7.58	12.64	13.07	12.14	21.86	51.40	6	39.97	6
West Lambeth	156 754	6.03	5.68	4.88	6.97	12.38	15.17	13.81	23.12	49.92	7	39.43	7
Islington	157 522	6.59	5.77	4.29	7.38	12.88	12.62	13.56	16.91	47.42	8	38.68	8
Bradford	328 952	5.66	7.66	2.70	6.76	13.48	14.91	10.77	14.08	44.14	9	35.75	10
Newham	209 128	5.15	7.15	3.00	7.81	12.68	18.11	9.17	26.60	43.40	10	34.84	12
North Manchester	143 779	6.94	6.30	3.23	8.25	17.39	13.01	9.42	4.04	42.22	11	35.01	11
Central Birmingham	177 271	5.72	6.77	2.94	5.79	16.44	15.88	10.55	20.09	41.51	12	33.83	13
Wandsworth	185 259	6.10	5.84	3.93	5.91	10.57	14.26	11.52	22.74	36.07	13	30.10	15
Hammersmith and Fulham	144 616	7.01	5.11	3.80	6.45	11.10	14.72	13.46	15.27	36.07	14	31.76	14
Lewisham and North Southwark	313 748	6.38	5.66	3.80	7.56	10.95	11.38	10.93	13.92	33.89	15	28.23	16
Bloomsbury	115 428	10.18	4.23	2.81	6.14	10.19	11.86	17.22	10.99	32.00	16	35.79	9
East Birmingham	203 881	5.24	6.69	2.38	6.67	16.71	16.78	7.73	15.83	30.82	17	24.91	17
Liverpool	503 721	5.72	5.92	2.82	8.69	19.83	11.96	8.49	1.68	30.59	18	22.89	19
Rochdale	211 003	5.46	7.08	2.85	6.50	12.87	11.00	9.10	5.11	29.23	19	22.32	20

identifying underprivileged areas. The values of the UPA scores (and of the eight variables which make up the scores) of the electoral wards of districts in England and Wales can be obtained from the Department of General Practice, Lisson Grove Health Centre, London NW8 8EG, by sending a request with a reply paid A4 size envelope.

THE 1987 WHITE PAPER ON IMPROVING PRIMARY HEALTH CARE SERVICES

The Acheson Report (LHPC, 1981) on primary health care in London put forward 115 recommendations for improvements that could be introduced. These included suggestions such as a retirement age of 70, later reducing to 65, for general practitioners. This and most of the other recommendations were not well received by general practitioners as a body and very few changes were made as a result of the report. There was some development of academic departments of general practice in London and improvement grants for upgrading practice premises were increased in some Family Practitioner Committee (FPC) areas. However, in spite of the paucity of action, there was a change in the climate of opinion. That there are problems for primary care in inner city areas came to be generally accepted (which was not the case previously): the evidence in the Acheson and other reports was consistent and conclusive. The difficulty has been getting helpful changes agreed and implemented. The 1987 White Paper (DHSS) may be more successful than previous reports. For instance, the question of a retirement age for general practitioners is one which, with the passing of six years since the Acheson Report and changing attitudes in the intervening period, will now in all probability be implemented.

The general principles of the White Paper are that the resources devoted to primary health care are to rise in real terms, additional revenue will be raised and a strategic shift in emphasis will be implemented. This will be aimed at making services more responsive to consumers' needs and giving them more choice, raising standards of care, promoting health and preventing illness. Although there are reservations over the method of funding the changes (such as the introduction of charges for eye-testing) and a lot of the necessary details are as yet missing, overall there is a good chance that many of these objectives will be met. The consultation process following the Green Paper which was published in April 1986 showed that people are particularly interested in accessible, effective and sympathetic primary health care services: prevention and health promotion: more information: the needs of the elderly and the problems of deprived inner city and isolated rural areas. Many of these problems have been tackled in the recommendations that have been made. There is, however, a suggestion that the capitation element of general practitioners' remuneration may be increased as a proportion of their total income. This, if carried too far, could take us back to the problems of the earlier capitation system. Much depends on the actual details of the implementation of the proposals.

THE WHITE PAPER RECOMMENDATIONS WHICH ARE SPECIFICALLY DESIGNED FOR, OR WILL BE PARTICULARLY HELPFUL IN, INNER CITIES

1. The introduction of an inner city 'deprived areas allowance'. This will presumably be paid to general practitioners working in the areas which are identified as being 'deprived', although the method of determining which these areas are is not spelled out. This is an important recommendation because it means that NHS general practitioners working in deprived areas with lower list sizes will be able to receive a gross income equal to that of general practitioners in other areas for an equivalent workload. The need for them to do non-NHS work should be decreased. As the minimum number of hours per week which a general practitioner must work and the minimum number of patients needed to receive allowances in full are both to be increased, this should ensure that this payment only goes fully to general practitioners with list sizes above these minima, with fairly large NHS workloads.

2. A registration fee for preventive work will be paid for those over 5 years of age when they first register with the NHS. This could be helpful because inner city areas have a higher turnover of patients. If the fee were each time a patient registered with a new general practitioner this would encourage acceptance of patients for whom there may be a large administrative workload when they register. This would include, for instance, homeless families and people living in hostels who often have

extensive psychiatric histories. In these cases there is a lot of work trying to trace the past medical histories from previous general practitioners and hospitals as their general practitioner notes are often lost because of their high mobility.

3. Differential and increased cost rent allowances will be paid for inner cities and arrangements will be made to make funds available for these developments in deprived areas if private sector funds are not available. This recommendation, if fully realized, could help to improve general practitioners' premises in deprived areas.

4. There will be a modification of the Medical Practice Committee (MPC) rules based on local information, especially in inner cities. This could mean that more general practitioners are allowed to practise in inner city areas if they are needed, even though the area list size may be lower than average. This recommendation will only work if the 'deprived areas allowance' is also brought in, because otherwise general practitioners working in these areas with lower list sizes and generally higher expenses will find that they will need to take non-NHS work to boost their incomes and there will be a return to the status quo.

5. The introduction of a system more related to medical and social needs and creation of new vacancies where workloads are high in relation to list sizes are further recommendations related to that in 4 above. This opens the way for varying the MPC rules to take account of the factors which increase the workload or pressure on the services of general practitioners and community nurses as measured by the UPA scores. Again, for general practitioners, it will be important to use this recommendation in conjunction with the 'deprived areas allowance' for the reasons given in 4 above.

6. A retirement age of 70 for general practitioners (possibly being reduced to 65 at a later date) will have a large effect in some inner city areas. The proportion of general practitioners aged 65 or more in some inner city districts in 1983 is shown in Table 6.4, together with the proportion practising single-handed. The national average proportion of general practitioners aged 70 or more is 2% and aged 65 or more is 5%. Table 6.4 shows that these figures are considerably higher in some districts, which are mainly in Inner London. Leeds Western, Central Birmingham and Brighton districts and nine other London districts also have more than twice the national average of general practitioners aged 65 or more. The vacancies created when these elderly general

Table 6.4   Proportions of Single-handed and Elderly GPs, 1983

District	% GPs aged 65 +	% GPs single-handed
Victoria	25	46
Bloomsbury	23	40
Paddington and N. Kensington	20	36
Tower Hamlets	19	22
Hampstead	18	41
West Lambeth	17	32
City and Hackney	16	36
Liverpool	15	17
Average for England	5	13

practitioners retire will give an opportunity for FPCs to build up primary care teams providing the types of services which are encouraged in the White Paper.

7. Removal of the present restrictions on the numbers of ancillary staff who may be employed (currently two per general practitioner) would give the opportunity for greater support for primary care teams in deprived areas. The wording of the recommendation also implies that the control of the total number of ancillary staff will be at FPC level and FPCs would effectively be cash limited regarding this aspect of their reimbursements to general practitioners. If these cash limits were to vary according to the level of deprivation this recommendation could be used to help deprived areas.

8. Making FPCs responsible for establishing group practices in deprived areas and also for making improvements in premises in these areas is another of the recommendations. Since FPCs became independent authorities in their own right on 1 April 1985 (as they were between 1946 and the reorganization of the NHS in 1974) they have taken a greater role in managing and planning their services. Setting specific goals for FPCs related to making these improvements in deprived areas (for the first time ever) combined with the recently expanded role of FPCs may prove to be a great help for inner city primary care. It should make it possible for FPCs to concentrate on developing primary care teams in good premises in inner cities – one of the key recommendations of the Acheson Report and also a separate recommendation of the White Paper.

9. The establishment of a fund to improve the standards of pharmacies in deprived areas should help to ease some of the difficulties which pharmacists also face as a result of practising in inner cities.

RECOMMENDATIONS NOT LIMITED TO DEPRIVED AREAS WHICH COULD BE HELPFUL IN INNER CITIES

Brief details of these are:

1.   More funds for FPCs.

2.   The number of general practitioners is expected to rise and the average list size to fall.

3.   The encouragement of a safe, effective and economical prescribing policy and the appointment of specially trained medical officers to promote better prescribing practice.

4.   Support for the training of medical students in general practice. Most departments of general practice at medical schools are in inner city areas.

5.   Postgraduate education for isolated and single-handed general practitioners.

6.   The introduction of a new postgraduate education allowance.

7.   Extension of the training of general practice professional staff.

8.   More women are to be encouraged to enter and stay in general practice.

9.   Increased development of computers and information technology in general practice.

10.   Remuneration for minor surgery could help to reduce referrals to hospital for relatively minor problems such as removal of warts and sebaceous cysts which can be dealt with in a well-staffed and equipped practice.

11.   Social workers working from the same premises as general practitioners can help to improve communications between social workers and primary health care workers. This is important in many instances such as child abuse cases.

12.   Direct reimbursement for interpreters and link workers in the surgery is particularly helpful where there are high proportions of ethnic minorities.

13.   Financial support for experiments in voluntary peer review may gradually lead the way to continuous assessment of

the standards of practice, including clinical care, of general practitioners.

14.   Doctors with abnormally high or low rates of hospital referral will be invited to take part in an assessment to help them make effective use of hospital services.

15.   Alignment of the FPC planning system with that of the hospital and community health services.

RECOMMENDATIONS WHICH ARE PARTICULARLY PATIENT ORIENTATED

1.   Making it easier for patients to change their general practitioner when they have not changed their address.

2.   Provision by FPCs of comprehensive information about practices.

3.   Encouraging practices to produce practice booklets for patients.

4.   Involving the public in changes which are made.

5.   FPCs will monitor the performance of general practitioners.

6.   Consumer surveys of samples of the population regarding the services provided.

7.   Services to be provided at more convenient hours for the patient.

8.   Introduction of informal conciliation procedures and easier complaints procedures.

RECOMMENDATIONS WHICH WILL PARTICULARLY HELP HEALTH PROMOTION

1.   FPCs to promote and evaluate health promotion policies.

2.   Provision of incentives for immunizations. It is important that any incentive payments take account of the greater difficulties that there are in achieving good immunization levels in inner city areas. (Jarman B. *et al* 1988).

3.   Remuneration for comprehensive regular care for the elderly.

4.   A registration fee for preventive work for those over 5 years.

5.   Development of suitably trained general practitioners to develop health surveillance of the under-fives.

6.   Cervical and breast screening and life-style advice (smoking, alcohol, diet and exercise) based on general practice.

7.   Payment of the basic practice allowance will depend on carrying out health promotion activities.

SUMMARY

The problems of inner city areas both for the people living there and for those providing primary care services for them have been discussed. It is shown that there is a way of assessing in which geographical areas these problems are likely to be most pronounced. There have been many reports which have analysed these problems and come forward with proposed changes designed to lead to improvements. Little as yet has been done. However, the 1987 White Paper on improving primary health care brings together many of the previous proposals and makes recommendations which could be both helpful and acceptable to those whom they most concern.

REFERENCES

DHSS (1981). *The Primary Health Care Team*. Report of Joint Working Group of the Standing Medical Advisory Committee and the Standing Nursing and Midwifery Advisory Committee (Chairman: Dr W. G. Harding). London: HMSO.

DHSS (1986a). *Primary Health Care: An Agenda for Discussion*. Cmnd 9771. London: HMSO.

DHSS (1986b) *Neighbourhood Nursing – A Focus for Care*. Report of the Community Nursing Review (Chairman: Mrs J. Cumberlege). London: HMSO.

DHSS (1987). *Promoting Better Health*. Cm 249. London: HMSO.

Hughes J. and Roberts J. (1980). Problems in the Development of London's Community Nursing Services. Project Paper **25**(3). London: King Edward's Hospital Fund for London.

Jarman B. (1981). A survey of primary care in London. Occasional Paper **16**. London: Royal College of General Practitioners.

Jarman B. (1983). Identification of underprivileged areas. *British Medical Journal*, **286**, 1705–9.

Jarman B. (1984). Underprivileged areas: validation and distribution of scores. *British Medical Journal*, **289**, 1587–92.

Jarman B., Basanquet N., Rice P., Dollemore N., Leese p.(1988). Uptake of Immunisation in District Health Authorities in England. *British Medical Journal,* **296**, 1775–78.

London Health Planning Consortium (1981). Primary Health Care in London. Report of the Primary Health Care Study Group (Chairman: Professor E. D. Acheson). London: DHSS.

OPCS (1986). *General Household Survey, 1984.* London: HMSO.

Royal Commission on the National Health Service (1979). The Report. Cmnd 7615 (Chairman: Sir Alec Merrison). London: HMSO.

Suggestions for further reading in addition to the above:

Abel-Smith B. (1976). *Value for Money in Health Services.* London: Heinemann Educational.

Allsop J. and May A. (1986). *The Emperor's New Clothing.* Family Practitioner Committees in the 1980's. London: King Edward's Hospital Fund for London.

Cronin A. J. (1937). *The Citadel.* London: Gollancz.

Honigsbaum F. (1979). *The Division in British Medicine.* London: Kegan Paul.

7

Mental Health

MATTHIJS MUIJEN and JULIA BROOKING

MENTAL DISORDERS

The effects of the environment on mental health

There is considerable evidence for a relationship between mental health and the physical and psycho-social environment (reviewed by Freeman, 1984). However, the nature of the link is far from clear and research in this area has produced equivocal results. The aetiology of psychiatric disorders is still poorly understood and it is probably futile to search for single causative agents. In addition, mental illness is not a homogenous concept and different disorders have widely varying aetiologies. In general, there is increasing recognition that many disorders are caused by a combination of factors, resulting from complex interactions between genetic predisposition, biological abnormalities and environmental influences throughout life.

Inner city living has been shown in numerous studies to be associated with high rates of mental disorder and other forms of social pathology. From the early work in the 1930s to the present day, the excess of schizophrenia in the deprived cental areas of big cities has been repeatedly confirmed (see review by Hare, 1982). In recent large-scale epidemiological studies in Britain and the United States the prevalence rates of a range of mental disorders and psycho-social problems have been found to be consistently higher for inner city residents than for people living in suburban or rural areas.

However, epidemiological data reflect only the level of a disorder, but do not explain its causes. The direction of the relationship between mental illness and inner city residence is uncertain and two competing, but not mutually exclusive, explanations are frequently cited.

One view assumes that an adverse environment itself contributes to the development of mental disorder. This 'social causation explanation' (Faris and Dunham, 1939) postulates that the stress of living under conditions of disadvantage increases vulnerability to emotional disorder. The link is therefore environmentally rather than individually determined. If correct, this view has obvious implications for remedial action to improve the quality of the urban environment to prevent or reduce its harmful effects. This might include urban renewal, rebuilding and relocation schemes. In contrast, the 'social selection' or 'social drift hypothesis' (Gruenberg, 1961) proposes that people who are affected by psychiatric morbidity tend to move down the social scale, clustering in deprived inner city areas where demands on them are less. In this model the locality is not seen as influencing the development of the disorder, but simply lacks the social structures that would make the deviant feel unwelcome and offers cheap single accommodation and opportunities for casual work.

This debate has continued unresolved for decades and it is probable that both processes operate simultaneously, albeit to different degrees in different circumstances and for different individuals. For example, social causation is well established in the case of depressive disorders, whereas social drift is thought to be particularly relevant to schizophrenia.

Research in this area is further complicated by methodological difficulties in case identification. Many early epidemiological studies used service utilization as their criterion of morbidity. However, this inevitably reflects availability, convenience and acceptability of services and referral patterns, as well as actual prevalence and incidence rates.

Features of inner city deprivation associated with mental disorder

The single feature of inner city life which has most commonly been found to be correlated with mental disorder is that of low socio-economic status. Indeed, Brenner (1979) described this as the single most consistent feature in the field of psychiatric epidemiology. Dohrenwend and Dohrenwend (1974) concluded that a higher rate of psychiatric symptoms was to be found among the poor and was associated with their experience of severe and frequent stresses especially in the urban environment.

Working-class people frequently have to cope with stresses without the financial and educational resources and social supports available to middle-class people. Summarizing results over a long period, Dohrenwend *et al* (1980) reported that low socio-economic status was particularly related to high rates of schizophrenia, personality disorder, depression and severe non-specific distress. This pattern has been observed repeatedly in American and British studies.

Low social class and poverty are typically accompanied by a range of problems, such as unemployment, single parenthood, divorce, high rates of birth, family deaths, physical morbidity, poor education and low intelligence. As these indicators of social deprivation are so frequently clustered together, it is impossible to disentangle how, if at all, they differ in their contribution to the development of mental disorders. This is further complicated by the immense variation in the ways that individuals respond to stressful life events. Significant mediating variables may include genetic and biological constitution, previous life experiences, general emotional health, vulnerability and personality, and social networks, including the existence of social support and confiding relationships. Mental and physical breakdown is rarely associated with a single major negative life event, but more usually results from chronic stress produced by a series of stressors, which individually may be insignificant, but which together over a prolonged period result in increased susceptibility to breakdown.

Sociological research has described the essential difference between urban and rural life as involving different qualities of inter-personal relationships associated with different types of social structures. The social problems of cities include heterogeneous and highly mobile populations, fragmentation of families and social networks, low participation in community activities such as church-going and high crime rates. The lack of coherent, identifiable and stable social structure underpins the stability of a society and was described by Durkheim (1897) as 'anomie', a major determinant of suicide. In Edinburgh, Buglass and Duffy (1978) found population mobility and overcrowding to be consistently associated with high rates of suicide and parasuicide.

Deprived inner city areas contain a high proportion of members of ethnic minorities and numerous studies have found increased rates of mental disorder among minority groups (see review by Cox, 1986). Schizophrenia is commonly found in young West Indians and they are noticeably over-represented among compulsory admissions to psychiatric hospitals, being frequently referred by the police or family rather than by general practitioners. Paranoid states have been found to be high in immigrants who speak the native language poorly, and who have insufficient contact with others of their own cultural background. Other studies have found a failure to diagnose and treat minor mental disorders, including depression. Parasuicide rates are higher in Jamaican immigrants to Britain than in those remaining in their country of origin (see review by Burke, 1986). Transcultural pyschiatry is in its infancy and the causes of these findings are little understood. Discussing reasons for high breakdown rates in immigrants Rack (1986) offers two possible explanations. One concerns the stress of migration itself, with separation from the familiar environment and the need to adjust to the social and political attitudes of the new country. The other is that migrant groups may contain a disproportionate number of people predisposed to mental instability. Stonequist (1937) described the dilemma of 'marginal man', stranded between two cultures, unable to identify fully with either, an inherently stressful position. To these must be added the experience of racial prejudice and lack of understanding between mental health professionals and patients from different cultural backgrounds.

Factors in the physical environment may be associated with stress, although it seems unlikely that structural factors are such important determinants of mental well-being as social factors. High rates of vandalism and mugging, whether real or imagined, increase fear, isolation and alienation and inhibit people from going out to meet others. Overcrowded housing reduces the ability to regulate the nature and frequency of social interaction and high rise flats contribute to difficulties in supervising children, restriction of social interaction and lack of territorial markers and defensible space. Reviewing the literature on the effects of noise, Monahan and Vaux (1980) concluded that excessive noise could decrease affiliative and helping behaviour, increase aggression and contribute to tension-related illness. Environmental pollutants and toxic wastes, produced by dense traffic, can also have negative effects on psychological and emotional functioning and are more common in big cities.

Mental disorders and social pathology

The whole range of major and minor mental disorders are encountered in inner city psychiatric practice. Downward social drift is likely to account for at least some of the high rates of schizophrenia, alcoholism, drug addiction and personality disorders. The stresses of inner city life itself can explain some of the prevalence of depression, the social causes of which were elaborated in a series of classic studies by Brown *et al.* (1978). They see depression as related to major losses, such as losing one's home or a significant relationship, as well as major difficulties such as overcrowding, physical deprivation, noise and lack of security of tenure. All these problems were more common in working-class than middle-class women. Vulnerability factors were also identified, such as lack of support from social relationships and low self-esteem. This model is compatible with another influential theory of depression. Seligman (1975) has produced evidence that depression is brought about by uncontrollable events which lead the individual to believe that responses are ineffective in obtaining the desired result. Lack of control over the vagaries of life is inevitable in people living in profoundly deprived circumstances.

City living is also associated with substantial amounts of deviant behaviour, manifest in forms of social disturbance such as delinquency and crime, disordered or broken family relationships, sexual deviation and addiction. Many of these problems cannot be described as mental disorders, although they often come to the attention of the psychiatric services and may have considerable aetiological significance both for the people engaging in deviant behaviour and for others around them.

THE PROVISION OF PSYCHIATRIC SERVICES

Range of services

The inner cities with their high prevalence of psychiatric morbidity demand a comprehensive network of services, ideally offering care to diverse groups varying from relatively minor anxiety states or problems in daily living (e.g. examination stress, fear of flying) to chronic major psychiatric illness (e.g. chronic schizophrenia). In the United Kingdom no single model of inner city psychiatric services exists but many different approaches are being used to serve essentially the same population. The community-care models of Lewisham and Nottingham differ considerably from the hospital-based service in Camberwell. Availability of essential facilities such as day-hospitals, day-centres, work units and drop-in centres vary widely, as do the range and numbers of professionals employed, such as community psychiatric nurses, psychologists, occupational therapists, social workers and psychiatrists. This can reflect as much the efforts and interests of the health services as those of local authorities and voluntary organizations, all of whom spend much of their resources on the chronic patients.

What can easily be forgotten is that the great majority of people suffering from psychiatric problems will never be in contact with the specialist services but instead consult their general practitioner. Even if patients do eventually see a psychiatrist, they almost invariably are referred by their general practitioners, and the system relies on their skills in recognizing symptoms and identifying needs. Therefore, any description of psychiatric services should start with primary care.

Psychiatry in primary care

The importance of the general practitioner is illustrated by the finding that they only refer 5.5% of patients they recognize as suffering from a mental illness to the psychiatric services (National Morbidity Study: HMSO, 1979). If they were to refer even another 1% of this group, an insignificant proportion of general practitioner attenders, the psychiatric service would collapse.

But do most people consult their general practitioners when they suffer from psychiatric symptoms? Community studies suggest they do. Brown and Harris (1978) found that 68% of their depressed women in the community had consulted their general practitioner, a proportion confirmed by other studies. Factors which seem to relate to mental-health consultations are severity, life-events, loneliness and female sex.

A second requirement for general practitioners to function effectively in managing psychiatric disorders is illness-recognition. The variation in the diagnosis of psychiatric illness between general practitioners is remarkable. Goldberg and Huxley (1980) in their survey of mental illness in the community reported ranges as wide as 0 to 90% for general practitioners, while psychiatrists tended to find a prevalence of about 30% among general practice attenders. The differences among general practitioners tended to depend more on their own characteristics rather than on differences in the prevalence of psychiatric illness. Accuracy was correlated with interview techniques such as good eye contact, sensitivity, the ability to clarify, confidence and high academic ability. Patient characteristics which could determine the detection of psychiatric illness were severity of symptoms, middle age, familiarity with the general practitioner and female sex.

Patients referred by general practitioners to the psychiatric services suffer more often from severe conditions or are psychotic, young, well-educated, unmarried, men or separated, divorced and widowed women. Older general practitioners refer more often than their younger colleagues. Urban practices refer more often than rural ones, which seems to be due to distances from the services rather than deprivation (Goldberg and Huxley, 1980).

The liaison of general practice with other disciplines will lead to an improvement in and a wider variety of services for patients and learning opportunities for both general practitioners and the mental illness specialists.

ATTACHMENT AND LIAISON SCHEMES

The role and training of mental health professionals

Psychiatrists, nurses, psychologists and social workers are increasingly establishing close links with general practices. In an attachment scheme the mental health worker is based at the practice, and will see clients who can be referred either by the doctor or from other sources, such as social workers, home helps, etc. A liaison scheme means that a general practice is regularly visited and cases are discussed, with occasional interaction between mental health workers and patients. In the liaison model the emphasis is placed on advice and teaching. The objective of the scheme is to bring in specialists at the earliest stage in a setting the patients find non-stigmatizing and convenient. All of the professions involved bring their own expertise from the traditional hospital settings to the surgeries. These developments are still in their infancy, but are likely to become of more importance with the growth of community psychiatry. Ideally the different professions would collaborate at primary-care level, but this is not yet the rule.

It is inevitable that mental health workers are able to provide only a limited service in primary care settings. The high number of general practice attenders with psychiatric problems means that specialists have to make decisions about their priorities because resources are limited. The population suffering from serious mental disorders are referred to the specialist services via out-patient clinics, crisis-intervention teams, day hospitals or hospital admissions where they will be assessed by a psychiatrist or other members of the mental health team. Although this implies that many people suffering from psychiatric problems never see a mental health specialist it also means that specialists assess and treat those with the most severe symptomatology. This may be appropriate as many primary-care attenders do improve over time, often spontaneously, while attenders of specialist services require more intensive and long-term care.

As yet there are few opportunities for mental health professionals to share multi-disciplinary education in community psychiatry, but this would be a valuable future development, given the existing blurring of roles and the need to improve communication and coordination among the various professional groups. Although increasing numbers of community psychiatric nurses take post-registration courses, there is doubt about the effectiveness of the existing training. For example, Wooff et al. (1988) found no differences in work practices between community psychiatric nurses who had undertaken specialist post-registration training and those who had not. The Community Psychiatric Nurse Association argues that specialist training should be mandatory, but given the increasing emphasis on community care, it can equally be claimed that the basic training should prepare nurses and other mental health workers to practise in all settings, not just in hospitals.

The psychiatrist

Psychiatrists use both attachment and liaison models. In Nottingham, Tyrer (1984) transferred some of his out-patient clinics to a primary-care setting in a deprived inter-city area. The large majority of patients were referred by the general practitioners, but a few were seen following discharge from hospital. Most patients suffered from neuroses (52%) and 15% from a psychosis, characteristics more similar to a psychiatric out-patient clinic than general practice. Advantages of the primary-care clinics were that patients preferred them, 19% said they would not have attended the hospital clinic, and better communications with general practitioners resulting in improved continuity of care. Also suggested was a reduction in hospital admissions, although at the time many other changes were taking place in the psychiatric services which may have contributed to this.

Experiences from liaison schemes indicate that a couple of hours of discussion a month between psychiatrists and general practitioners can mean a greatly improved contact between the services.

The community psychiatric nurse (CPN)

Psychiatric nurses in Britain began to work outside hospitals in the 1950s with the establishment of the first CPN service at Warlingham Park Hospital in Surrey. At that time the work consisted of after-care of discharged schizophrenics, specifically supervising drug regimes. Rapid expansion of community psychiatric nursing began in the 1970s and most health districts now have access to a CPN service.

A variety of patterns of service have developed. Most commonly CPNs work in the community all the time, but some have both in-patient and community responsibilities for the same patients. This has the advantage of giving continuity of care during admission and after discharge, but is administratively complicated, with the demands of ward work frequently taking priority over community work. Most early CPN services were established as part of consultant-led multidisciplinary psychiatric teams, but there has been an increasing trend to attach CPNs to general practice as part of primary care teams. Inevitably, work location influences the nature of the work, with primary care CPNs caring mainly for patients who are not referred to psychiatrists, such as those suffering from neurotic and personality disorders and relationship problems. In contrast CPNs attached to psychiatric teams work mostly with patients suffering from major mental disorders, such as schizophrenia. Both types of attachment are valuable as they meet the needs of different patient populations, but lack of clinical supervision is a serious problem for general practice attached CPNs, who may be the only psychiatric specialists in the primary care team. The majority of CPNs are generalists, dealing with a variety of clinical problems, but specialism is increasingly common. Some CPNs have taken advanced training to work with particular patient groups, such as children, adolescents or the elderly; others specialize in particular types of intervention, such as behaviour therapy, family therapy, crisis intervention or rehabilitation.

The role of the CPN is immensely varied, encompassing all aspects of psychiatric nursing practice, as well as expanding into work conventionally carried out by other professionals such as general practitioners, psychiatrists and social workers. There has been much discussion about role overlap between CPNs and social workers and it is noteworthy that the expansion of CPN services parallels the decline in availability of specialist psychiatric social workers. There is also some role overlap with health visitors and district nurses.

Most CPNs work on a one-to-one basis, typically in patients' homes, supplemented by contact with patients' families. The role can include the whole range of social, psycho-therapeutic, behavioural and physical aspects of nursing, including supervising and monitoring drug and other treatments. CPNs may provide practical assistance with accommodation and employment as well as promoting social interaction and they give support, education and advice to families and others involved with their patients. Because of the autonomous and highly responsible nature of the work, most CPNs are registered mental nurses at charge nurse grade, but some staff and enrolled nurses work in the community.

There have been many descriptive studies of CPN services, but few evaluations of their clinical efficacy. In a prospective controlled trial in Tooting, London, Paykel et al. (1982) (see also Paykel and Griffith, 1983) compared a consultant-based CPN service with routine out-patient care. Subjects were 99 patients suffering from chronic neurotic, affective and personality disorders, predominantly middle-aged, working-class women, who were randomly assigned to one of the two conditions and followed up over 18 months by researchers not involved in treatment. Treatment was given as clinically indicated, with the out-patients seeing either a consultant or junior doctor at a clinic and the CPN group being seen mainly in their own homes and receiving a mixture of supportive counselling, supervision of medication and occasional use of other regimes.

The findings of this study support the continuing development of community psychiatric nursing in that there were no significant differences between the two groups of patients over time on symptoms, social role performance and degree of family burden. CPNs achieved a higher number of discharges than psychiatrists and patients' satisfaction with treatment was significantly higher in the CPN group, with nurses rated as significantly easier to talk to, more interested, pleasant and caring than psychiatrists, an effect which increased over time. Although CPN care was initially more expensive, over the whole study period it was less costly than out-patient treatment. It is important to note that the CPNs were working in multi-disciplinary teams, receiving advice and support from psychiatrists, so this study is not a comparison of the efficacy of two professional groups, but rather of two modes of service. It is likely that beneficial features of the CPN service were its flexibility in the frequency of contract; the location of treatment in the home rather than a clinic; the duration of contacts which lasted an hour on average, compared with fifteen minutes for an average out-patient consultation; contact with patients' families; and its stability in that patients saw the same nurse over a prolonged period, whereas the psychiatrists were in rotating training posts.

The social worker

In inner city areas, with a high proportion of social problems such as single mothers, housing shortages and high crime rates, many general practice consultations would be more appropriately dealt with by a social worker. However, because of the shortage of social workers, they are of necessity mainly occupied with their statutory responsibilities such as child-care. Therefore they are rarely able to work in settings other than the area office.

In the primary care setting, referrals to social workers are mostly for practical problems, such as finances or housing, but they see more patients with mental illness or emotional problems than their colleagues at area offices (Corney, 1984). Social workers have key roles in supporting the mentally ill, such as offering practical support, staffing day-centres and hostels and representing the patient under the Mental Health Act. Because their role in mental health care is unique and specialized, this should be reflected in a specialized training. However, since the implementation of the Seebohm Report in 1971 the social work training, lasting two years, has become generic (non-specialized), with trainee social workers receiving a basic training not specifically related to their future work. Four post-qualification psychiatric courses exist, but relatively few social workers attend these.

A change in the 1983 Mental Health Act stipulates that those social workers who are involved in the involuntary admission of patients to a psychiatric unit have to be 'approved'. Local authorities are supposed to design training courses which would provide the social workers with a working knowledge of mental illness and the intricacies of the Mental Health Act. To achieve these aims fully, however, the course should be more comprehensive and extensive than it is at present.

Many social workers pursue their personal interests, and take courses in areas such as family therapy. This expansion of their traditional role and skills is likely to make them more effective, although there is a risk of loss of their own expertise and excessive overlap with other professions.

The psychologist

Clinical psychologists have many appropriate skills to manage general practice attenders. Kincey (1974) suggested the following problem areas as particularly suitable for psychologists:

1. Problems of anxiety and stress;
2. Habit disorders;
3. Educational and occupational difficulties or decisions;
4. Interpersonal, social and marital problems; and
5. Psychological adjustment to problems stemming from physical illness or other significant life events.

This represents such a large proportion of patients that psychologists have to prioritize and this is facilitated by the emergence of specialist nurses who have received advanced training in behaviour therapy. Also, some social workers are well qualified to deal with many of these areas. At present the numbers of clinical psychologists are too low to provide a significant primary-care service. Primary-care seems to be a natural setting for psychologists with their interest in early intervention and mental health in contrast to psychiatrists who tend to concentrate on mental illness.

The interest of psychologists in community care has developed since the implementation of the Trethowan Report in 1977 which stated that psychologists should offer a district service led by a psychologist rather than psychologists being members of hospital psychiatry departments as they had been before. This meant that psychology had to redefine its own role which it seems to have done successfully. In 1981, a postgraduate qualification was made an obligatory condition of becoming a clinical psychologist in the National Health Service. Areas of training as listed by the British Psychological Society include assessment, research and management (Liddell, 1983).

COMMUNITY CARE

Traditionally, psychiatric treatment has been delivered in the mental hospital often many miles from the patient's home. This dates back to the 1850s when large asylums were built outside the inner cities. Only in the last three decades have psychiatric units been established in general hospitals with the idea of integrating mental health care in the community. In contrast to the past when the mentally ill were treated solely in asylums without any other provisions, the general hospital units aim to be part of a comprehensive service, including facilities such as out-patient clinics, day hospitals and day-centres. The emphasis has changed gradually from the hospital as centre of treatment to the community. Mental health workers now attempt to provide care for people outside hospital and admission is increasingly considered only as the last resort.

The experience that skills learned in hospital do not generalize to the patient's home environment and the fact that no correlation is found between behaviour in hospital and behaviour in the community (Fontana and Dowds, 1975) implies that effective treatment needs to be offered at the place where those skills have to be applied. In hospital settings the emphasis is on remission of symptoms, whereas community care concentrates on practical skills required for everyday life.

The essence of community care is offering patients individualized care which maximizes functioning in their own environments while minimizing dependency on services. A fine balance needs to be struck between minimizing dependency with the risk of neglect and offering constant care in residential settings. This latter approach to care can cause institutionalization as easily in hostels and group homes as in large mental hospitals.

Community care as an alternative to hospital care

The role of the hospital is multifarious, including psychiatric, medical and nursing care, temporary accommodation, food, occupation, social contacts and respite to both patients and their relatives or friends. Especially in inner city areas with the high prevalence of social problems, the non-psychiatric components are important. Many patients are admitted for a crisis and stay in hospitals for long periods in spite of only moderate symptomatology because they have no person or place to return to and no appropriate facilities, such as hostels, are available. They become attached to staff and other residents and industrial therapy takes the place of rehabilitation or employment. This leads to hospitals becoming home and place of work simultaneously with an exclusion of the outside world. If in addition staff do not allow initiative and patronize their patients, institutionalization will be reinforced and may become irreversible. However, many studies have indicated that by transferring the locus of care from hospital to less restrictive placements, such as hostels or independent accommodation, the development of dependency can be avoided or partly reversed.

Two different target groups can be identified who may benefit from community care. The first group is the chronic mentally ill who have often spent many years in asylums and are due to be transferred back into the community as a result of hospital closures, termed de-institutionalization. In contrast, the second group is the seriously mentally ill, marginally living in the community, as often as not on their own, who require regular brief admissions for relapses, termed the revolving door syndrome. Eventually it is likely that these two groups will fuse, as the community group will need increasing care, including placements in the facilities built for the ex-hospital patients, while the chronically ill will make demands on services initially meant to prevent hospitalization for the more acute and younger group.

Comprehensive community care requires a wide range of services. Not only should it provide accommodation with varying degrees of support but the other functions of a mental hospital cannot be ignored. Day-hospitals are necessary for psychiatric and medical care, day-centres for short- and long-term skills training, drop-in centres for social contacts, a range of industrial rehabilitation units suited to the variable work needs of patients and trained staff for home assessments. Nevertheless, even where these facilities exist, hospital beds have to be available for crisis-intervention and some special need groups such as forensic patients and a gradually diminishing group of high dependency patients who are presently unwilling and unable to live outside hospital. All this means that the decentralization of psychiatric care will involve the building and running of many small units. This has implications for efficiency both in terms of cost and coordination of various services.

Most studies comparing alternative forms of care with standard hospital treatment included both new patients and patients well known to the services. A large amount of literature suggests that many alternatives to hospital benefit these patients clinically and socially, frequently saving some costs too (Kiesler, 1982). The alternatives include day hospitals, hostels, foster homes, patients' own homes, and combinations of settings. Treatment models also vary from crisis intervention and family therapy to rehabilitation.

One example is the project which was started in Sydney in the early 1980s (Hoult et al, 1983). All patients in need of admission, except those with addictions and brain damage, were randomly allocated to an experimental community group or a control hospital group. All patients suffered from serious mental illness (50% schizophrenia), and people on hospital orders or presenting with violence or suicidal ideas were included. Eight staff consisting of nurses, social workers, a psychologist, an occupational therapist and a part-time psychiatrist, looked after the sixty community patients. Following randomization to community care, patients were assessed by the staff. If at all possible they were taken home, and received intensive treatment. Care and support was provided to patients and relatives, seven days a week, twenty-four hours a day, with an on-call service during the night. Hospital admissions were used for the shortest possible period only if patients were very disturbed. During the one-year project, the community patients were regularly visited, with the aim of improving their functioning in their own environment, where it would benefit them most.

Patients in the experimental community group and the control hospital group were independently evaluated at baseline and at the end of the twelve months. The results showed that the community-care group had a significantly superior clinical outcome: only 40% had needed admission, as compared with 96% of the hospital group. If admitted, the duration was only a third of that of the hospital group.

Only 8% of the community group, and about 51% of the hospital group, had needed more than one hospitalization. Admission increased the probability of further admission, a finding shown in many other studies. In addition, the satisfaction of patients and relatives was much higher for community care. Particularly successful was the outcome of new patients in the community group; the chronic patients showed similar small improvements with either community care or hospital care. Impressive is the consistency between studies on all these findings, despite considerable methodological differences. No controlled study has found a superiority of hospital treatment over community care in any of its forms (Kiesler, 1982).

The possible advantages of community care should not be exaggerated. All experimental groups still showed considerable symptomatology and disability in spite of their comparative improvements. The effectiveness of the community services is supported by the fact that after their withdrawal and the reintroduction of standard services the patients gradually lost their acquired gains and the differences between experimental and control groups disappeared.

Cost-benefit analysis indicates that some savings can be achieved by providing community care, although these savings are small. However, capital costs are rarely included, and initially, at least, good quality community care should not be expected to save money.

Practical experiments in the United States

Since the early 1960s community mental health centres have become part of the psychiatric services in the United States. The intention of these centres was to achieve a shift in care from hospital to the community by providing comprehensive and continuing care for the mentally ill. However, a shift in ideology from care to prevention developed in many centres. Staff in some community centres hoped to prevent the onset of serious mental illness by offering crisis intervention to people with problems, the 'unhappy but healthy', at the expense of the long-term mentally ill, who suffered neglect. For example, the proportion of community centre patients suffering from schizophrenia has been reported as 10%, while 20% were diagnosed as 'not mentally ill'. Parallel with this was the reduction of medical staff, with an increase in numbers of psychologists and social workers. Mental illness became defined as a social problem, which required social intervention. Because of this move away from care for the mentally ill, federal health programmes discontinued their funding, and insurance companies followed this by refusing to reimburse non-medical attendances at community centres. As a consequence morale dropped, with an increase in staff turnover, resulting in poor care (Langsley, 1980).

Fortunately this decline was reversed by the government providing guidelines which had to be satisfied before funding was approved, and which led to the development of some outstanding community services. One such service is the experimental project comparing home with hospital care in Madison, Wisconsin, which after proving its effectiveness has continued as a regular service for ten years (Stein and Test, 1980). It offers a comprehensive community based service for the mentally ill. At present it consists of four units: a crisis intervention service; a mobile community team for the population which needs long-term care; the out-patient services for the less needy patients; and a day-centre. Patients enter the system at the crisis intervention service, where they are assessed. If only a short-term intervention seems necessary, patients will be dealt with by the crisis team, but otherwise they will be referred on to appropriate segments of the service. In turn, all services can request the crisis team to manage a well-known patient temporarily, using their specific expertise. Flexibility is an essential part of this system. Because it is recognized that a community approach can only function if admissions are monitored and limited, the crisis team is given the task of assessing all patients who may need admission. If admission is avoided the crisis service has a responsibility to provide alternative care. Good use is made of imaginative projects such as foster beds and crisis hostels. In the American system where the private sector provides a substantial proportion of the health care private patients may be admitted directly and offered follow-up care based on psychotherapy. Since community care has been demonstrated to be superior to hospital care in most studies, it is somewhat ironic that patients who can afford private treatment receive hospital admission followed by psychodynamic therapies, while those who cannot are provided with community care. It is hoped that treatment allocations in the United Kingdom will be based on outcome studies rather than on financial imperatives.

Key principles of community care

For community care to be a real and positive alternative to hospital based care, it has to fulfil strict criteria of quality. It should provide a comprehensive and equitable service, caring for minor and major psychiatric disorders and offering a range of treatment facilities. In addition community care faces the inherent disadvantage of decentralization which makes good communication between different and often remote parts of the service a priority. Guidelines put forward in the United States (Turner and Ten Hoor, 1978) specify that an adequate community service must provide ten functions:

1. Identification of the target population and the staff to offer appropriate services.
2. Support with social services.
3. Crisis intervention with a range of facilities, including hospital.
4. Psycho-social rehabilitation, including assessment, training on living skills in the natural setting, work, housing and social skills.
5. Continuity of care for as long as necessary.
6. Medical and mental health care.
7. Support to relatives, friends and employers.
8. Involvement of community members.
9. Protection of client rights.
10. Case-management to ensure the coordination of different services.

Case managers, or key workers, play a central role in community care. Their function is based on the idea that each patient requires individual care which may change over time. Case managers have the responsibility to assess their patient's needs, develop an individualized care plan, coordinate the various services involved, monitor the quality of those services, and evaluate progress. Objectives of case-management are the enhancement of the quality and continuity of care, the enhancement of accessibility and accountability, and the improvement of efficiency (Intagliata, 1982).

Without case-workers various health workers can be involved with the same patient, unaware of the overlap in services, and not coordinating their care. This is not only inefficient, but can also be dangerous; for example, when patients receive several prescriptions for medication.

However, there are also potential disadvantages to a case management system, both to staff and patients. Staff have to accept a considerable responsibility, including the emotional dependency of their patients. This means high levels of stress, and can lead to staff burn-out. Ways of diminishing this pressure are careful key-worker allocations, the sharing of tasks, and mutual support within the team. Most mental health teams consist of a mixture of professions, and background and training of staff is not always taken into account when a key worker is selected. This can result in additional staff pressures, such as inexperienced nurses having to manage difficult social problems, while social workers may have to offer generic care to their clients. Rationalization of patient load not only provides a better service for the patient, but also alleviates pressures on the staff and enhances their feelings of being valued. The disadvantage to patients can be a dependency on a single member of staff. Difficulties are often experienced when the key worker is on holiday or changes jobs.

Eventually a model of care should develop which provides a compromise between the individual case-management approach and a shared team approach, making full use of staff's expertise, while providing individual continuing care to patients.

THE FUTURE OF PSYCHIATRIC CARE IN THE INNER CITIES

Financial

At present psychiatric care in the United Kingdom is largely based on a loose collaboration between health authorities and local authorities, without any national guidelines. Although this offers maximum flexibility, it also means that quality varies as a consequence of different priorities and large differences in health spending. Hospitals are financed by the health services, but many community facilities such as day-centres and hostels have to be to be financed by the local authorities.

The twenty most deprived districts in the United Kingdom, according to the Jarman indices (Jarman, 1983) are all large inner city areas, while the twenty least deprived districts are all suburban or rural. This has important implications for the financing of community care in the inner cities, as most inner city local authorities have to make provisions for the relatively large number of mentally ill people living in their area. This is reflected in the extreme differences in health care expenditure between inner city areas and suburban areas. For example, some Inner London boroughs, e.g. Wandsworth and Westminster, spend over £6 per head of population on mental health care, while one London suburban borough (Redbridge) only spends 49p a head. Local authority budgets are restricted by political decision. For example, many inner city areas are rate-capped. These restrictions do not exist for residential care, which is fully financed by central government, and unrelated to expenditures of local authorities. Patients living in private, often profit-making residential homes, are fully paid for by social security. Clearly, local authorities will find it difficult to finance comprehensive community care given their limited budget, but central government sponsors private residential care without financial limitations. This situation is described by the Audit Commission for Local Authorities (1986) as the 'perverse incentive against community care'.

It has been suggested that money for mental health care could be transferred from the health authorities to the local authorities. At discharge of a patient from hospital to a community placement, a yearly sum of money is freed by the health authority, which can amount to £12 000. This is called 'endowment money'. This sum follows the patient, and can be used by the local authority for the provision of services. The health authority will remain responsible for medical care. The local authority would not be given any finances for services required by people who never needed hospital care, which is a further disincentive against the development of community resources. The Griffiths Report (1988) suggests a clarification of these respective responsibilities by the appointment of a Minister of State for Community Care. Objectives, priorities and standards will have to be laid down, and local authorities should be provided with the funds to match their responsibilities. If implemented, this would result in a marked change in health care.

Services

In spite of financial hurdles, interesting projects have developed
locally in the United Kingdom. A Mental Health Advice Centre
opened in Lewisham, offering a walk-in facility and a crisis
intervention team as an alternative to out-patient clinics and
hospital-admission respectively. Since the start of the project the
demand on out-patient appointments was much reduced, but
numbers of hospital admissions were not affected. The severity
of patients' conditions seen at the two facilities was very
different; 38% of the crisis team patients but only 8% of the walk-
in clinic patients were psychotic (Boardman and Bouras, 1988).
This difference between patient groups resulted in the use of
different management techniques. Counselling was offered to
50% of new walk-in patients, but only to 16% of the crisis
patients. In contrast 25% of crisis patients and only 2.5% of walk-
in patients were admitted to a psychiatric hospital. This illus-
trates how a variety of services is needed to provide the most
appropriate care for different groups of patients.

It is likely that future services will be based on relatively small-
scale developments such as the Lewisham Centre. Care has to be
taken that patients will not be lost, falling in the gaps between
the various services. Such a model can only be effective if each
centre knows its own role in the whole organization. Individual
centres need to be well defined, aiming to serve a specific target-
population, such as young schizophrenics or people with marital
difficulties, within a comprehensive service.

Before the large-scale implementation of community services
begins, it is important to assess the efficacy of the different
models of care that are available. For example, in South South-
wark a project is evaluating the feasibility of home-care for the
seriously mentally ill in a deprived inner city area (Marks et al,
1988). If projects like this prove to be successful, many hospital
admissions may be prevented, and resources could be transferred
to the community. However, caution is necessary as unvalidated
decisions based on enthusiasm rather than research could adversely affect the services provided to many people well into the
next century.

CONCLUSIONS

Inner city psychiatry may not be essentially different from the practice of psychiatry in other settings. Nevertheless, this chapter has shown that factors associated with the high levels of social deprivation found in inner cities are likely to contribute to the development and course of both major and minor mental disorders as well as other indicators of social pathology. Although there is no simple causal relationship between the inner urban environment and mental breakdown, it is clear that social factors are relevant to mental health in a variety of ways. They may contribute to breakdown itself, to the likelihood of recovery and relapse and are relevant to the ways in which services could be organized.

In considering the provision of psychiatric services for the inner city, this chapter has discussed the need for the range of services, including hospitals, day-centres and a variety of community facilities. Good psychiatric practice is characterized by its diversity, encompassing all types of psychiatric interventions, according to the problems identified. These can range from prevention, short-term crisis intervention and medium-duration treatments, through to long-term support and rehabilitation.

This chapter has deliberately avoided discussion of the relative advantages and disadvantages of particular theoretical approaches, recognizing that behavioural, psycho-dynamic, social and biological perspectives all have something to contribute to the development of services for the inner city. There is no one theory of community psychiatry. It is premised on a recognition that patients' problems must be understood and treated in the context of their social environment, including the family, domestic circumstances, work and other social and economic factors. The needs of families and/or friends, who provide most of the care and support for patients, must be as much the focus of attention as the needs of the patients themselves.

Given that most psycho-pathology is and inevitably must be dealt with by the primary care services, the importance of the general practitioner has been emphasized. Community psychiatry cannot simply reproduce the patterns of hospital treatment, from which general practitioners are excluded. Specialist community psychiatric teams must work closely with primary care teams, rather than merely taking over patients. This change in emphasis will require sensitivity in developing mutually supportive relationships with the existing primary care services. Community psychiatry is administratively complex and some of the bureaucratic and financial difficulties have been considered. Closer liaison between health and social services is essential if good practice is to develop.

This chapter has emphasized that inner city psychiatry should be a multi-disciplinary endeavour, with members of all mental health disciplines contributing their specific areas of expertise and knowledge. This is potentially problematic as there is no clear consensus about role boundaries between different members of the team. The blurring of roles inherent in the 'key worker' system may be desirable, but it raises questions about decision-making, leadership and accountability in teams. It also brings into question the traditionally separate training received by the different psychiatric professions. As key workers, nurses are attractive to policy makers because they are cheaper to employ than most other mental health professionals, but salary differentials may become difficult to justify if different team members do essentially the same work and can be shown to be equally effective. There are also ethical and political issues in the decisions about which professionals act as key workers for which patients. There may be a risk of these decisions being made on social class lines, with more patients in the inner cities being treated by nurses, but more patients in the affluent suburbs being treated by doctors.

A number of examples of innovative community projects in inner cities in Britain and elsewhere have been cited but these remain the exception rather than the rule. This chapter has argued for the further development of community psychiatric services, but this change would require a massive reorientation of attitudes among psychiatric professionals. Despite the community-care policies of successive governments and the closure of many large mental hospitals, there is still a widely held view that community services exist to support a hospital-led service, rather than the view that hospital beds should exist to support a predominantly community-led service, using admission only when patients cannot be maintained in their own homes. For most general practitioners, contact with consultant psychiatrists is largely confined to referrals and liaison over occasional domiciliary visits. In most parts of Britain, CPNs and to a lesser extent social workers are the sole psychiatric specialists who have any significant community base. The establishment of CPN services, although important, is just one very small step towards the ideals of comprehensive community psychiatric care, provided by multi-disciplinary community psychiatric teams, working in close collaboration with primary care teams, social services and voluntary agencies.

REFERENCES

Audit Commission (1986). *Making a Reality of Community Care.* London: HMSO.

Boardman A. P. and Bouras N. (1988). The Mental Health Advice Centre in Lewisham. *Health Trends,* **20,** 59–63.

Brenner M. H. (1979). Influence of the social environment on psychopathology: the historic perspective, in Basset J. E. (ed.) *Stress and Mental Disorder.* New York: Raven Press.

Brown G. W. and Harris T. (1978). *Social Origins of Depression.* London: Tavistock.

Buglass D. and Duffy J. C. (1978) The ecological pattern of suicide and parasuicide in Edinburgh. *Social Science and Medicine,* **12,** 241–53.

Burke A. W. (1986). Racism, prejudice and mental illness, in Cox J. L. (ed.). *Transcultural Psychiatry.* London: Croom Helm.

Corney R. H. (1984). The mental and physical health of clients referred to social workers in a local authority department and a general practice attachment scheme. *Psychological Medicine,* **145,** 137–44.

Cox J. L. (ed.) (1986). *Transcultural Psychiatry.* London: Croom Helm.

Dohrenwend B. P. and Dohrenwend B. S. (1974). Psychiatric disorders in urban settings, in Caplan G. (ed.). *American Handbook of Psychiatry,* 2nd edn, Vol 2. New York: Basic Books.

Dohrenwend B. P., Dohrenwend B. S., Gould M. S., Link B., Neugebauer R. and Wunsch-Hitzig R. (1980). *Mental Illness in the United States: Epidemiologic Estimates.* New York: Praeger.

Dunham H. W. (1961). Social structures and mental disorders: competing hypotheses and explanations. *Milbank Memorial Fund Quarterly,* **39,** 259–311.

Durkheim E. (1897). *Le Suicide: étude de sociologie.* Published in English in 1951. Glencoe: Free Press.

Faris R. E. L. and Dunham H. W. (1939). *Mental Disorders in Urban Areas.* Chicago: Hafner.

Fontana A. F. and Dowds B. N. (1975). Assessing treatment outcome and adjustment in the community. *The Journal of Nervous and Mental Disease,* **16,** 221–30.

Freeman H. L. (ed.) (1984). *Mental Health and the Environment.* Edinburgh: Churchill Livingstone.

Goldberg D. and Huxley P. (1980). *Mental Illness in the Community.* London: Tavistock.

Griffiths R. (1988). *Community Care, agenda for action.* London: HMSO.

Gruenberg E. M. (1961). Comments on 'Social structures and mental disorders. Competing hypotheses of explanation', by Dunham H. W., in *Causes of Mental Disorders: a review of epidemiological knowledge 1959.* New York. Milbank Memorial Fund. Cited in Lorion R. P. and Felner R. D. (1986). Research on mental health interventions with the disadvantaged, in Garfield S. L. and Bergin A. E. (eds) *Handbook of Psychotherapy and Behaviour Change* (3rd edn). New York: Wiley.

Hare E. (1982). Epidemiology of schizophrenia, in Wing J. K. and Wing L. (eds). *Psychoses of Uncertain Aetiology. Handbook of Psychiatry,* **3.** Cambridge: Cambridge University Press.

Her Majesty's Stationery Office (1979). *Morbidity Statistics for General Practice.* Second national study 1971–1972. Studies on Medical Population Subjects, No. 36. London: HMSO.

Hoult J., Reynolds I., Charbonneau-Powis M., Weekes P. and Briggs J. (1983). Psychiatric hospital vs community treatment: the results of a randomised trial. *Australian and New Zealand Journal of Psychiatry,* **17,** 160–7.

Intagliata J. (1982). Improving the quality of community care for the chronically mentally disabled: the role of case management. *Schizophrenia Bulletins,* **8,** 655–79.

Jarman B. (1984). Validation and distribution of scores. *British Medical Journal,* **289,** 1587–92.

Kiesler C. A. (1982). Mental hospitals and alternative care. *American Psychologist,* **37,** 349–60.

Kincey J. (1974). General practice and clinical psychology – some arguments for a closer liaison. *Journal of the Royal College of General Practitioners,* **29,** 337–40.

Langsley D. G. (1980). The community mental health centre: Does it treat patients? *Hospital and Community Psychiatry,* **31,** 12, 815–19.

Liddell A. (1983). *The Practice of Clinical Psychology in Great Britain.* Chichester: Wiley.

Marks I. M., Connolly J., Muijen M. (1988). A controlled cost-effectiveness study of community-based versus standard in-patient care of serious mental illness. *Bulletin of the Royal College of Psychiatrists,* **12,** 22–3.

Monahan J. and Vaux A. (1980). Task force report: the macro environment and community mental health. *Community Mental Health Journal,* **16,** 14–26.

Paykel E. S. and Griffith J. H. (1983). *Community Psychiatric Nursing for Neurotic Patients: The Springfield Controlled Trial.* London: Royal College of Nursing.

Paykel E. S., Mangen S. P., Griffith J. H. and Burns T. P. (1982).

Community Psychiatric Nursing for neurotic patients; a controlled trial. *British Journal of Psychiatry*, **140**, 573–81.

Rack P. H. (1986). Migration and mental illness, in Cox J. L. (ed.). *Transcultural Psychiatry*. London: Croom Helm.

Seligman M. E. P. (1975). *Helplessness*. San Francisco: Freeman.

Stein L. J. and Test M. A. (1980). Alternative to mental hospital treatment: 1 Conceptual model, treatment program and clinical evaluation. *Archives of General Psychiatry*, **37**, 392–7.

Stonequist E. V. (1937). *The Marginal Man* (reissued 1961). New York: Russell and Russell.

Turner J. C. and Ten Hoor W. J. (1978). The N.I.M.H. Community Support Program; Pilot approach to a needed social reform. *Schizophrenia Bulletin*, **4**, 319–48.

Tyrer P. (1984). Psychiatric clinics in general practice. An extension of community care. *British Journal of Psychiatry*, **145**, 9–14.

Wooff K., Goldberg D. P. and Fryers T. (1988). The practice of community psychiatric nursing and mental health social work in Salford: some implications for community care. *British Journal of Psychiatry*, **152**, 783–93.

8

Old age

FIONA ROSS

> Old age can only be understood as a whole: it is not solely a
> biological but also a cultural fact.
>
> (de Beauvoir, 1972, p. 20)

INTRODUCTION

This chapter focuses on old age in the inner city, using some
sociological theories of ageing as a framework. The size of the
elderly population and their needs is reviewed with particular
emphasis on being old and female, isolated, single, homeless, and
a member of an ethnic minority group. Some of the negative
effects of inner city living are considered; for example, poverty,
threat of crime, violence and abuse. Service provision is discussed in terms of use, appropriateness, unmet need. In the light
of current policies to promote community care some important
issues are considered; for example, the role of the informal carer,
and augmented care. Finally the problem of developing a
strategy of coordinated care to old people in the inner city is
addressed.

THEORETICAL PERSPECTIVES ON AGEING

There are a number of emergent and contrasting perspectives on
ageing that have different academic origins. They are to an
extent related, with common themes and complementary ideas.
This section is an overview, with a particular focus on some key
sociological theories that can be used to enhance understanding
of ageing in the inner city.

The biological model has been influential in policy and practice. This depicts ageing as a process of continual and inexorable decline, with the onset of pathological changes in physical health. Deterioration of mental health is part of the same process, and important links can be made with loss of role and status. Thus ageing is viewed in terms of physical and mental degeneration, with increasing incidence of illness, and dependency.

> I'm an old woman now
> And nature is cruel,
> 'Tis her jest to make
> Old age look like a fool.
> The body it crumbles
> Grace and vigour depart.
>
> (Elder, 1977, p. 8)

The concern of much sociological research has been the social context of old people's lives, in particular housing, health, poverty and isolation. There are two opposing sociological approaches to ageing. First acquiescent functionalism, which attributes the problems of the elderly to the difficulty of adjusting to becoming old. The work of Cumming and Henry (1961) on disengagement is important in that it has had an influence on policy and practice. The substance of this theory is that as people grow older, they experience role loss and diminished social interactions, resulting in disengagement from social involvement. Given that this was a single unreplicated study, using American middle-class subjects, its impact in terms of ideas and policy in Britain has been remarkable. It reinforces the biological model of ageing, justifies a *laissez-faire* and passive response from practitioners, and condones the 'warehousing' and institutionalizing of the elderly that denies individuality and discourages initiative.

The alterntive sociological explanation to acquiescent functionalism sees old age in the context of class, occupation and gender issues. It is known as structured dependency. This provides the argument that old age and dependency is a social construction (Walker, 1982), and that society reinforces class, gender and income differentials in old age. Furthermore, the response of professionals in health and social services is determined by social position and assumptions learnt through training and socializa-

tion. Therefore professionals may enhance or reduce dependence
of old people through their attitudes and practice.

The life history and biographical approach has origins in both
psychological and sociological traditions. It takes account of how
old people see and value their own lives and the meaning of
social events. Johnson (1986) states that what emerges is a
distillation of their lives, which provides the basis of their self-
esteem, self-image and future.

> I'll tell you who I am ...
> I'm a small child of ten,
> with a father and mother
> brothers and sisters who
> love one another ...

(Elder, 1977, p. 7)

In summary, these ideas have been influential and continue to be
so on policy and practice. The stereotype of old people as a
homogenous group, and a problem category, has been the
underpinning for ageism, labelling, institutionalization and an
absence of innovation in care. Structured dependency helps to
clarify the structural factors that shape policies, services, and the
professional and personal response to old people. The biographical approach seeks to understand old people as individuals,
enabling a positive view of the future through focusing on what
is important and meaningful. In the rest of this chapter these
ideas will be discussed in relation to specific issues in the inner
city.

PROFILE OF OLD AGE AND THE DIMENSIONS OF NEED

It is well known that demographic changes taking place now will
lead to a considerable increase in the number of very elderly in
the United Kingdom's population. Although the retirement age
population will remain steady, it increased to 9 million in 1984
from 8.9 million in 1981 (OPCS, 1985). It is expected that up
until the end of the century, there will be a continuing and
dramatic growth in the very old, and that those aged 85 years
and over will make up 12% of all people of pensionable age in
2001 compared to 7% in 1981.

Old people are not only becoming older, the majority (97%) live in the community in private households, and most are female. In the inner city the number of old people has been rising as the population as a whole has fallen. High social mobility and migration from the inner city have meant that families have fragmented, leaving old people behind. Living alone and its consequences of isolation, lack of support and risk are commonly associated with old age. While the estimated proportion of old people living alone varies, there is a consistent trend that it is higher in the inner city, and the figure increases sharply with age. Although living alone does not necessarily imply social isolation or indeed loneliness, among this group there are those at risk because of physical incapacity, bereavement through loss of a spouse, or because of deprivation factors in the inner city.

WOMEN AND OLD AGE

Women outnumber men by a ratio of 2:1 among those aged 60 years and over. The proportion rises with age, and twice as many women as men live alone. It has been argued that the feminist movement has ignored the needs of women in old age, and that social policy has largely failed to distinguish between the needs of the sexes. Popular mythology of ageing incorporates stereotypes of old women that are usually derogatory, exposing them to the double rejection of ageism and sexism.

It is not untypical for old women living in the inner city to be living alone, possibly isolated, experiencing feelings of loss and abandonment as partners die, and families move away. Added to this is the pain of seeing their own children now also elderly in poor health or dying. As well as being alienated from the outside world, and loved ones, these women may themselves be in poor health, have reduced mobility, and living below the poverty line, because they are less likely to be eligible for occupational pensions. In addition, many frail elderly women are still caring for others, with little help from the services. There is some evidence that criteria based on gender are used, although seldom explicitly, in allocation of services to old women compared to old men (Parker, 1985).

An interesting study that set out to explore the realities of daily life and support relationships from the perspectives of older women living alone has been reported by Evers (1984). She identified two extremes: the 'active initiator', who sees herself in control in spite of relying on others for help with basic activities; and the 'passive responder' who depends on others to organize and structure her life in spite of having the capacity for greater independence. Evers develops the argument beyond that of the individual old woman's adjustment to ageing, to the assertion that attitudes to ageing and dependency are influenced by past experience, social circumstances, and rehearsed methods of coping. This has obvious implications for professionals to accurately identify how the individual perceives her dependency in order to make appropriate interventions.

POVERTY

The association of poverty and old age has long been established. The poverty of old people in the inner city reflects class, housing, deprivation and ethnic factors. Elderly people from the lower social classes are generally less likely to have earnings as a major source of income, and are mostly dependent on state pensions and other social security benefits. The basic pension in April 1987 was £39.50 for a single person, and £63.25 for a couple. Age Concern argues that almost half of all pensioners cannot live on their pension alone, and therefore have to claim supplementary benefit. In 1983 almost 1.7 million persons over pensionable age (about 17% of the total) were receiving supplementary benefit. In the same year pensioners also accounted for one-fifth of exceptional needs payments (Family Policy Studies, 1986). Further, about half of all elderly black or Asian people receive supplementary benefit, as they are much less likely to receive any kind of pension. Another indicator of poverty is housing. In general, old people are less likely to be owner occupiers, and more likely to live in rented, local authority accommodation or in private rented and unfurnished rooms. The latter typically includes housing stock with the most inadequate amenities; for example, elderly people living alone are three times more likely to have no inside lavatory as a non-elderly household.

The evidence suggests that the old in Britain are poor, and there is an expectation that impoverishment is an inevitable part of ageing among the working class. The problem of poverty is compounded in that as many as 35% of old people do not claim their benefit entitlement.

The introduction of the new benefits system in April 1988 will affect old people in a number of ways. The individual allowances for diet, incontinent laundry, and heating have been abolished, and replaced by income support. Secondly, the new housing benefit will be calculated using new rules and taking into account savings. The pensioners' lobby has criticized this move as being a penalty on thrift, and claim that at least 250 000 old people will lose benefit altogether. The new cash limited social fund replaces single payments. It is discretionary, and with the exception of the community care grant and funeral payments, is recoverable by the State.

ETHNIC ELDERS

The 1985 Labour Force Survey shows that only 3% (66 000) of the non-white population is of pensionable age compared with 19% of the white population (OPCS, 1986). The needs of ethnic elders have been passed over for a number of reasons, which include the assumption that this numerially insignificant group of old people are cared for by the extended family. The policy of integration is now challenged by research and pressure groups, because it is seen to lead to cultural isolation and the provision of inappropriate services. This section discusses three main aspects of ethnic elders: the shared concerns of all old people; the specific needs of old people from ethnic groups; and the implications for services in the inner city.

Old blacks, as well as old whites, living in the inner city are disadvantaged in terms of poor housing, low income, and the experience of living in a bleak and alienating environment. (The term 'black' is used here to describe people of both Afro-Caribbean and Asian descent.) In addition there is the possible threat to health and mobility, loss of the social networks associated with work, as well as facing an uncertain future. Superimposed on the devaluation of old age and living in the inner city is the experience of prejudice and discrimination. Old people from ethnic minority groups have come from different countries with different cultural, religious and social structures. Barker (1984) challenges the assumption that membership of ethnic minority groups is homogenous. He argues that the biographies of old people in many ethnic minorities are by definition often the histories of unusual people, unique to a particular point in history, and that their experiences are unlikely to have much in common with future generations who will neither have been pioneers nor have been brought to Britain as dependents in old age.

What, then, are the problems faced by these ethnic elders? Barker found in his study of ethnic elders in Manchester and London that the majority reported loneliness, and isolation, loss of role and dignity. Common problems identified were poor housing, low income, difficult access to health and social services, and feelings of powerlessness.

Blakemore's (1983) exploration of the effects of inner city living on Birmingham's old whites and old blacks (West Indians) is interesting in the insight it provides on the differential effect of the environment. Most of the old whites had spent all their working lives in the area, whereas the old blacks had arrived in migration waves of the 1950s. On the whole, the old whites were advantaged in terms of property ownership, and better pensions. However, old whites felt alienated and insecure in a neighbourhood most had grown up in. Old whites expressed feelings of helplessness in the face of rising crime and violence, whereas old blacks were more fatalistic. Some of the old blacks' dissatisfaction was channelled into a longing to go home.

The main conclusion of work in this area is that health and social care is often insensitive, limited and fails to offer an appropriate service tailored to individual ethnic need. The debate on what needs to be done has largely polarized between the lobby for integration and that of separate services. There are problems with both these approaches – integration, for example, in residential care means cultural isolation and rejection. On the other hand separation or segregation may lead to a second-rate service.

Most new initiatives for the elderly have come from the voluntary sector; for example, AFFOR (All Faiths For One Race) a multiracial resource based in Birmingham, which has made a number of innovations, including Asian meals on wheels, home helps, housing schemes, and promotes community action and self-help groups. There are some housing schemes that promote sheltered accommodation; for example, the Carib Housing Association in Kensington and Chelsea for elderly West Indians, and Aram House for old Asian men in Newham. In addition, special day clubs and resource/advice centres have been set up; for example, the Black Elderly Project in Wandsworth, which has Local Authority funding. The special needs of ethnic elders for housing has been studied by Age Concern (1984). This report identified a lack of awareness among service providers of housing needs and it recommended ethnic monitoring and closer collaboration between agencies.

The health services have also been slow to recognize ethnic needs. There is evidence that black elders tend to be unrepresented among health service users. Many of the factors that contribute to low uptake stem from service ethnocentrism, stereotypical views of black people, and inflexibility in the organization and delivery of care. Clearly there is a need for improvements in training, as well as management support and professional development.

THE SINGLE HOMELESS

The increase in single homelessness can be attributed to a number of factors, including the rundown of psychiatric hospitals, decline in the private-rented sector, unemployment, and increase in deprivation and poverty. The old are part of this, indeed they form an important part of the stereotype of the homeless old 'tramp' or 'dosser'. Blacher (1983) found that half the men in his study were alcoholics, and the majority had chronic illness or disability. The most frequent health problems were bronchitis and arthritis.

Blacher use an ethnographic approach to study the older single homeless in a night shelter in Plymouth. Although Plymouth does not share the core features of inner city deprivation his intrepretation of the meaning of vagrancy for these elderly has relevance. He makes the important conclusion that homelessness is not seen as an undignified and hopeless existence but as an expression of liberty. This value on independence is paradoxical, because their circumstances govern their lives almost entirely. Contrary to the myth that the homeless have an aimless existence, Blacher describes a daily routine that is often highly structured perhaps around the relentless need for alcohol. The older homeless tend to be less geographically mobile, more isolated, with a network of acquaintances, no real friends, and only a carrier-bag of possessions.

THE CARERS

The consequences of community-care policies, and the current vogue for efficiency, savings and focus on throughput, mean that old people are cared for longer at home, spend less time in hospital, and are discharged at an earlier stage of recovery. The ideology of the present government emphasizes the resources and energy available in the community, and policies over the last ten years have promoted the caring role of the family.

The research on informal carers has taken a new direction since the early seminal work of Peter Townsend (1957) on the family support networks of old people in East London. This study portrayed close-knit communities to which the old people contributed on the basis of gift exchange. The changes in the inner city over the last thirty years have resulted in an inevitable decline in family support, for reasons outlined earlier.

The current proliferation of studies on the informal carer comes from two main perspectives, which to some extent overlap. First the approach of the policy lobby has been to criticize the inadequate funding of community care. For example, studies carried out for the Family Policy Studies Centre (Parker, 1985) and the Policy Studies Institute (Nissel and Bonnerjea, 1982). The second important approach to this issue comes from feminists concerned with the way in which the caring role may restrict opportunities for women. The conclusion reached from this line of inquiry is that the majority of the estimated $1\frac{1}{4}$ million carers are women — daughters, wives, mothers, friends and neighbours. Nissel and Bonnerjea's case study of twenty-two families revealed that husbands rarely gave direct help to their wives with the care of a dependent relative, even when the wife was employed outside the home. Much of this work emphasizes the family burden of caring, and in particular the impact on women.

From both perspectives the burden of caring is often discussed in terms of the physical, psychological, social and financial costs. This separation is somewhat artificial, because of the links, for example, between physical and psychological well being. The physical demands from the duration of the caring episode, the time spent on caring tasks are likely to take their emotional toll. There is growing evidence that many carers have their own health problems, and that caring is stressful. Problems found to be stressful include the dependent's immobility, incontinence, mental changes, and sleep disturbance. The third consequence of caring is social isolation. There is some consensus from research that carers are isolated from help except in a crisis when families and services rally round. Finally the financial costs are considerable in terms of lost income and career opportunities, heating, laundry and equipment expenses, which are not compensated for adequately by benefits such as the attendance allowance and the invalid care allowance.

In summary, the nature of the task is continuous, exhausting and often frustrating, leading to expressions of despair such as: 'People don't want to know.' 'It is like looking after a child without the joy' (Nissel and Bonnerjea, 1982).

Feminist research has made an important contribution to defending the right of women not to be forced into a caring role through lack of an alternative. However, a limitation of this approach is that it perhaps exaggerates the issue of 'burden' and overlooks the subtleties of a relationship that is often not straightforward. A more helpful explanation is the concept of mutuality, which enables interpretation of the relationship in terms of giving and receiving. The motivation to care may be a mixture of obligation, responsibility, and love. There is little doubt that caring produces conflicts; for example, the sadness of seeing the slow deterioration and illness of a close relative, which brings with it the unfamiliarity of a changing relationship, role reversal, and the powerful, often opposing, feelings of love and resentment.

There are important implications of this work for the carers of old people in the inner city. Loosening of family ties and increased mobility means that the caring network is stretched. This is borne out by the number of frail spouses and increasingly ageing children looking after very old parents unsupported by younger family members, living in deprived areas, and in poor circumstances.

Services for carers have been criticized as inflexible and unimaginative, and not sensitive to individual needs. As Goodman (1985) notes there is an unfortunate assumption often made by professionals that the presence of a carer means that less input is required. Exceptions to this are often made if the carer is male. It is clear from the evidence that a new strategy for carer support must be formulated that crosses professional boundaries. The primary health care team has an important role to play and in particular the district nurse, often the 'linchpin and coordinator' of community care for the dependent elderly. If this is so then it is essential that she recognizes the support needed by families to continue caring, above all to give the 'listening kind' of help valued most by one group of carers (Nissel and Bonnerjea, 1982).

OLD-AGE ABUSE

The term 'granny battering' in general use and enjoyed by the media, reinforces the ageist and sexist stereotypes that all old people are little, old, defenceless ladies. Old-age abuse on the other hand is a term which suggests a link with child abuse, and puts the problem firmly in the family context. Eastman (1984) argues that the problem of old-age abuse is not yet recognized as such, it is unresearched, and the underlying factors poorly understood. A working definition describes it as systematic maltreatment, physical, emotional or finanical, of an elderly person by a care giving relative (Eastman, 1984, p. 23). One of the problems of this difficult area is defining the boundaries of abuse. Where does normal family conflict end, and abuse begin? For example, the tension, anxiety, and fatigue felt by a frail old lady caring for her dependent helpless husband may lead to frustration, anger, harsh words and perhaps withdrawal. The professional's dilemma is to identify at what point the conflict becomes damaging.

There is some evidence that dependency and disability are related to abuse. This on its own is an insufficient explanation and other factors may include the stress of caring; having other dependents, for example, children to look after; family friction; inadequate statutory support. Other predisposing factors may include vulnerability of the old person, lack of support and friendship networks, role reversal and low income. An assumption is often made that poverty is related to violence against old people. However, Eastman argues that there is little evidence to support this. His social work case material suggests that this multifaceted problem cuts across social boundaries, and is hidden deep within the complexities of physically and emotionally dependent relationships. The pain, guilt, and misery of the family dynamics that lead to abuse, leave more than just one victim.

The signs and manifestations of abuse that the professional must be alerted to include: bruising, sexual abuse, misuse of medication, recurring or unexplained injuries, physical constraints, malnutrition, and lack of personal care. Professional intervention for old people, suspected of being in an abusing relationship, is fraught with difficulties, because of the absence of clear guidelines on which to base practice. This is in contrast to the system for child abuse, which has at risk registers and a professional bureaucracy ready to go into action for suspected cases. Clearly, prevention of old-age abuse requires a multidisciplinary approach. Given that the district nurse has a potential role in reducing the stress of a caring relationship, then she has an important preventive role. However, clarification is needed on the implications for confidentiality, advocacy and the Law. Some of these issues, such as representation, procedures, and reporting have been recently addressed by Age Concern.

Old people may also be subjected to other sorts of violence, such as crime and victimization. It has been suggested that it is something of a myth that old people are more likely to be victims of crime than other age groups. This raises the question that if the elderly are undervictimized, why has this myth grown up? It is perhaps true to say that those most fearful of crime are not necessarily those who have experienced victimization. It has been found in Inner London that old people commonly feel it is unsafe to go outside, and especially at night. Thus the perceived threat of victimization may restrict the old person's life further and intensify the feeling of isolation and alienation. In recent years there has been an increase in the number of frauds and con tricks on old people, that have taken place within the home. This type of crime takes advantage of trust, and requires community vigilance to prevent.

HEALTH AND SOCIAL NEEDS

This section aims to look briefly at the information relating to physical and mental health of old people, and their social needs. The argument outlined earlier, that dependency is a social construction, has a bearing on the definition and the identification of health needs. Further, the interrelationships between physical, psychological and social needs are poorly understood. However, information on dependency is important, because it reflects need, and has implications for service provision.

In spite of the inequalities in health, which are reinforced in old age, the high use of health and social services, and the high incidence of long-term illness, research shows that most old people rate their health as good. For example, a community survey of old people in London found that 86% of the old, and 88% of the old old rated their health as excellent and good, in spite of disabilities (Copeland *et al*, 1986). This supports the findings of others, and fits with Evers's theory discussed earlier of the 'active initiators' and the 'passive responders'. Thus it may be that old people see their health in terms of what they are able to do within the constraints of their own lives.

The consensus from most studies is that in terms of mobility more old people have problems *outside* the home, than with mobility within the house, and that most people are not seriously disabled and are able to look after themselves. Copeland *et al* found that the incidence of depression in a random sample of old people registered with general practitioners in London was 17%. These diagnoses were made at a home interview by a psychiatrist, which may have identified milder cases. The same study identified 4% of cases with dementia.

SERVICES FOR OLD PEOPLE IN THE INNER CITY

Statutory, voluntary and private sectors provide a mix of health and social care, which rely on a variety of funding systems, care models, and combinations of professional and lay support. This section sets out to discuss service provision for old people in terms of use, appropriateness, and unmet need, and in the light of current policies to promote community care within a rationed service. It is impossible to examine in detail the full range of services in this chapter, therefore the focus will be on exploring the principles that underpin service delivery and the particular problems of the inner city.

The ideology of care

The health service in Britain was conceived and developed using the medical model of disease as its cornerstone. The dominant view of old people as a homogenous group, with the inevitable physical and mental defects of old age, has resulted in a negative stereotype, and the view that old people constitute problem categories. It is well documented that the main strength of the National Health Service has been to provide acute care, but its failure has been in terms of long-term care and prevention. To the extent that old people have required the interventions of acute medical care the NHS has provided appropriately. The growth of geriatric medicine has been slow, due to lack of funds and its low status in the medical hierarchy, but it has a key role in active assessment and rehabilitation. In addition many geriatric units now have day hospitals which provide a bridge between hospital and community, and services for the elderly mentally ill are growing.

A major trend in the policy response to the demographic changes has been the promotion of community care, and the identification of the elderly as a priority group. The rationale for the development of community care derives from the belief that institutional care fosters dependency and deprives individuals of self-determination. Linked to this is the rising expectation for health care, the challenge of intractable chronic disease, and the view that community care offers a cheaper option at a time of dwindling resources. It is against this background of economic recession and a growing demand for care, particularly from those groups for whom conventional medicine has little to offer, that official statements over the last twenty-five years have promoted the theme of community care. There are a number of problems with the implementation of this policy, including the loose definition and vague objectives which has suited the rhetoric of both main political parties; secondly, the opposition from power-ful vested professional interests to transfer of resources from the acute sector to the community; thirdly, community care and the needs of old people have less appeal than technological medicine to the public imagination and the media, and is thus a reflection of the negative stereotype that society has of old people. Finally, the concern with formal rather than informal care means that the burden of care increasingly falls on the family and women.

The gap between the political rhetoric and the reality of practice has been criticized in a number of recent reports; for example, the Audit Commission (1986), which led to the latest Griffiths Inquiry (Griffiths, 1988).

Use of services

It is well known that old people make more use of the health and social services than the average for other age groups, and the very old use them most of all. The problem of unmet need has been widely reported; for example, there is evidence that one-quarter of all old people do not receive visits from the social, health or welfare services and less than 20% go to social or day-centres (Hunt, 1978). Although it is difficult to know to what extent low uptake is due to unmet need or individual choice, there is little doubt that access to the health service presents more problems for old people. It is likely that use of services has also been affected by cuts in spending, which have forced health and local authorities to make uncomfortable decisions about priorities. At the same time it is the service providers at the sharp end of policy implementation who ultimately choose the priorities, and who play an important role in deciding who gets what and when.

Primary health care

The members of the primary health care team with a key role with old people are the general practitioner, district nurse, nursing auxillary, and the health visitor. It is well known that old people make frequent use of general practitioner services. The recent White Paper on primary health care reports that on average a general practitioner has five consultations per annum with each patient aged 65–74 compared with 3.8 for patients aged 5–64. For patients aged 75 or over the number rises to 6.3, which is reflected in high prescribing rates (DHSS, 1987).

The evidence suggests that the district nursing service only reaches a small proportion of the elderly population. Figures vary from 8% in a national survey (Hunt, 1978) rising with age to 20% of those 85 years and over (Bond and Carstairs, 1982). It is interesting to note in a study of service provision carried out by an Inner London borough, that although the elderly themselves considered a good primary health care service a priority only one-third of the sample was aware of the existence of the district nursing service, including 13 out of 34 housebound respondents (Campbell, Mitchell and Earwicker, 1981). This must indicate a demand for district nursing inadequately met. The district nurse has an important actual and potential contribution to make to the care of old people, including the well elderly. As well as the analysis of need, provision of care and support for old people in their own homes, residential care and sheltered accommodation, the district nurse is involved in health promotion, mobilization of professional and voluntary agencies, and the support of carers.

Health visitors also have a role in the support screening and health maintenance of old people, particularly the well elderly. However, the time spent by health visitors is variously estimated between 4% and 6% (Hunt, 1978; Strang, Craine and Acheson, 1983). Further, the number of visits to old people has decreased by 6% from 1979 to 1982. This is probably because of other pressures, such as child abuse. The health visitor has an important role in screening and health maintenance of old people.

Perhaps the most important feature of primary health care is the variability in facilities, staffing, and the organization of care. Delivery of care reflects geographical, class, and client group inequalities – particularly evident in the inner city. A point of relevance here is the staff shortages, high turnover, and stressful work experienced by community nurses in the inner city. This has implications for district nurses in that their care of old people tends to be reactive and pressurized. On the other hand, health visitors' work is caught up in complex family crises, and childcare problems. In most cases work with the well elderly is not a priority. Often for old people primary health care can depend almost entirely on the general practitioner with whom he/she is registered.

In spite of the unsatisfactory nature of the present system, primary health care does offer enormous potential for effective and holistic care for old people, which goes beyond dependency models of health and old age, and begins to foster independence and self-care. In order to achieve this primary health care, professionals need to work more closely together, as well as identifying and agreeing care objectives with their patients. Effective teamwork makes the assumption that professionals share a core of knowledge and further that this knowledge matches that of the patient. In an attempt to look at this I have completed a study that compared doctor and nurse knowledge of prescribed medication with their elderly patients. The findings showed that there were serious differences in knowledge. The discrepancies between doctors' and nurses' knowledge of their patients' drugs indicated inadequate communication and shortcomings in the medical records. If teams are to be coordinated and effective then they must have access to reliable clinical information. Although the role of teams in the delivery of patient education is relatively unstudied, there is a consensus that the multidisciplinary approach is the way forward. Sharing information with people and thereby challenging the traditional barriers between the health care system and the consumer is a key issue for primary health care.

Local authority services

Local authority services consist mainly of social services and housing. Social services provide day-centres, home-helps, meals-on-wheels, aids for daily living, as well as case work. It has been widely documented that only a small proportion of old people receive support from statutory domiciliary services and use day-centres. Although social service provision has improved, because of the growing numbers of old people, services are spread more thinly. This trend was confirmed by an Age Concern survey of services for the elderly in inner London: improvements in domiciliary services were insufficient when increased numbers of old, particularly the very old, and reduced family support was taken into account. For example: the household (that is the most dependent) rarely received services (Snow, 1981).

Residential care

Wilcocks (1986) estimates that 2% of the elderly population occupy residential homes. Current figures suggest that of these 56% live in public sector homes, 20% in homes supported by the voluntary sector, and 24% in private homes. It is interesting that the number of places offered by the private sector has increased by 10 000 between 1984 and 1985 alone, due to opportunities for funding through social security payments, and probably because of pressure on local authority provision. Grundy (1987) points out the paradox that the only real growth of provision for old people has been in private residential care, and that the ideological debate on this issue focuses on increased choice and commercial exploitation of old people. It is probably true to say that in spite of attempts to improve the design of accommodation and provide flexibility in living space, the residential life of older people remains predominantly public and collective, rather than private and individual (Willcocks, 1986).

Other problems of residential care include the increasing dependency of occupants, inadequate training and support of staff, poor coordination with the primary health care team and isolation from the surrounding community. An important and wider issue is the lack of flexibility and choice for long-term care, which reflects in part shortcomings in policy and professional practice.

Housing

Just over half of elderly couples, and 38% of older people living alone, are home owners. Forty-two per cent single elderly households, and just over half of old couples live in local authority housing. Although only 8% of the population live in private rented accommodation this includes a disproportionate number of old people (Wheeler, 1986). Only 6% of the elderly population live in sheltered accommodation. Inner city housing for old people in many ways reflects the deprivation and inequalities of old age. The problems of London are somewhat special in that the slum clearance and rebuilding following war damage, and the property boom, have resulted in the unique situation of old people living in rundown and neglected houses, cheek by jowl with the affluent middle classes.

It is now more widely recognized that there is a high proportion of owner occupiers living in unsatisfactory housing. There are a number of reasons for this, including the older nature of properties, low incomes and failure to apply for statutory improvement grants.

The main focus of housing policy over the last twenty years has been to promote sheltered accommodation, funded in the main by local authorities, sometimes housing associations and increasingly by the private sector (the latter mostly in the South-East of England where the market exists). While undoubtedly meeting a need, there are various problems with sheltered accommodation in that it creates age segregated housing, with little consideration of the views, and increasing frailty of old people. One of the main conclusions from the research on sheltered accommodation is that for some people they are there for want of a better alternative. There is little doubt that many old people move to escape loneliness only to find a greater alienation in unfamiliar surroundings.

Housing policy is beginning to shift from 'moving on' to 'staying put'. This involves various strategies initiated by Local Authorities and housing associations, including 'care and repair', advice on alterations, insulation, modernization. However, progress in this area is often limited by the lack of coordination between housing and social service departments in the Local

Authority, and structural separation between the public and private sectors.

INNOVATIONS IN CARE

A number of innovative approaches have been made to address some of the problems with service provision discussed in the previous section. There are many examples of 'good care' in the inner city and a few are described here.

Respite Care is increasingly offered by geriatric hospitals and residential accommodation to provide short-term care. There is some evidence that this has a measurable effect on reducing family stress.

Augmented home care schemes are often joint funded by a local authority and the health service, or funded by independent organizations such as Crossroads. The general aim of these schemes is to provide support in terms of personal and domestic help to the frail elderly, chronic sick, and the disabled at home and so prevent an otherwise inevitable admission to long-term care. A recent review of domiciliary services indicates that the impetus for innovation has come from local authority social services, voluntary agencies, and research initiatives; for example, the Age Concern programme for the mentally frail at Newham. Local authority schemes include alarm systems and services based on various types of personal care; for example, visiting wardens, home aides or neighbourly helps. The main thrust has come from the development of the home-help service to provide intensive, comprehensive personal and domestic care, which aims to promote rather than undermine existing lay helping networks. The emphasis is on flexibility, creating a service that will complement and integrate with other forms of community support. These developments have important implications for the primary health care team and in particular the extent to which there is role overlap with the district nurse.

A new and exciting innovation is the concept of the community-care centre recently set up in the London Borough of Lambeth. The aim is to provide support, care, treatment and rehabilitation from a multidisciplinary team, including family doctors, nurses, physiotherapists, and lay workers. The approach to care is individual, holistic, and attempts to build on the existing social and lay caring networks throughout. The centre has twenty beds as well as a day unit and facilities for use by community groups.

NEW DIRECTIONS

A major theme of this chapter has been to focus on the idea that old people are not a homogenous group with needs easily categorized. They have their own memories, experiences and outlook on the future. Even if some patterns and shared life views are discernible, policy makers need to be wary before prescribing care in a wholesale fashion. It is probably fair to say that many of those old white people in their eighties and nineties living now in the inner city have lived within the same area for most of their lives, and experienced poverty, hardship, and losses from two world wars, as well as being part of immense social change. There is something remarkable about their stoicism, pride and forebearance in a world that can be alien and hostile. As Doris Lessing puts it: 'They have already been felled several times, and picked themselves up, put themselves back together, each time with more and more difficulty, and their being on the pavement with their hands full of handbag, carrier bag, and walking stick is a miracle' (Lessing, 1983, p. 174).

This section sets out to discuss ways in which care for old people could be improved. The key policy of community care, which has received both support and criticism, has currently been subjected to a new reshape in the Griffiths Report. The recommendations include a new ministerial responsibility, and a lead role for Local Authorities in terms of financial control, and a coordinating function. Although the report is evasive about resources, in content it is radical and points to a way forward that deals with the thorny issues of collaboration and coordination. Even if the Government accepted the proposals, which is doubtful at a time when the role of Local Authorities is increasingly eroded, there is a lot more thinking needed on the implications for primary health care, community nursing and general practice.

It would be naïve to ignore the challenge that increasing privatization presents to old people. The present Government's enthusiasm for private health care ignores the uncomfortable fact that even if old people could afford the premiums the cost of long-term care would be prohibitive, resulting in a two-tier system.

A report that has made a considerable impact on community nursing is the Cumberlege Report (DHSS, 1986). The central message was to set up neighbourhood nursing teams to promote closer working relationships between health visitors and district nurses and to provide sensitive care to the consumer. While supporting the main thrust of the proposals it would seem that an unfortunate consequence of forging strong nursing teams is to make it less likely that energy will be put into developing links with other members of the primary health care team. It is interesting that many of the Cumberlege enthusiasts are in the inner city where there are particular problems with establishing primary health care teams. Some critics claim that Cumberlege has been interpreted as an excuse for another management reshuffle. However, in some inner city areas Cumberlege has been the necessary impetus for change and innovative ideas coming from district nurses and health visitors working together; for example, setting up health shops and initiating hypothermia campaigns.

Perhaps more fundamental than management reorganization is the need for change in professional attitudes. The roots and manifestation of ageist views were discussed earlier, but their pervasive influence throughout institutional and community care are undoubted.

> Our campaign for Annie is everything that is humane and intelligent. There she is a derelict old woman, without friends, some family somewhere but they find her condition a burden and a scandal and won't answer her pleas; her memory going, though not for the distant past, only for what she said five minutes ago; all the habits and supports of a lifetime fraying away around her, shifting as she sets a foot down where she expected firm ground to be ... and she, sitting in her chair suddenly surrounded by well wishing faces who know exactly how to set the world to rights.
>
> (Lessing, 1983, p. 162)

What then should be the proper focus of our care? Professional arrogance is no longer tenable. Rather this question leads to a discussion of the self-care debate. The self-care concept assumes the individual's integrity in decision making and subsequent actions that necessarily take precedent over professional values.

But this does not mean to say that self-care is mutually exclusive of professional care, or that professionals have a right to promote a version of self-care that means abandonment and isolation. Self-care, then, must be a shared activity between patients, professionals and families, and it must allow the old person control, autonomy and the right to participate.

The self-care approach has clear links with the biographical theory of ageing, because of the value attached to the individual's own interpretation of life. Further, it seeks to enhance autonomy, and self-empowerment, which may in fact conflict with professionally defined goals, as described in the case of Annie above. These life skills need to be nurtured, and preparation for retirement should begin early in terms of finding fulfilling leisure activities, alternatives to work, and developing meaningful social networks possibly through self-help groups. The role of the professional should not only aim to enhance individual strengths, and facilitate the development of new skills, but also identify ways of helping the consumer to define a relevant and appropriate service.

There is a recognized need for more information and improved communication between professionals and the consumer. There are frequent references in the literature of the importance of a team approach to the review of old peoples' needs. Successful teamwork depends on the patient or client being actively involved in care, and all team members sharing, and contributing fully to information and discussion.

In conclusion, the single most important idea developed in this chapter is the need to understand and address the needs of old people as diverse and individual. The tendency to stereotype and apply ageist theories and blanket policies has been criticized, and illustrated by the problems of ethnic elders, older women, and the informal carers. The ideology of care and the organization of services for elderly people are grounded in the medical model and crisis intervention. The challenge of the future must be to develop a truely collaborative framework, working across agencies, and together with the consumer to provide comprehensive and relevant care.

REFERENCES

Age Concern (1984). *Housing for Ethnic Elders*. Age Concern/Help the Aged Trust.

Audit Commission (1986). *Making a Reality of Community Care*. London: HMSO.

Barker J. (1984). *Black and Asian Old People in Britain*. London: Age Concern.

Blacher M. (1983). Elderly vagrants, in Jerrome D. (ed.), *Ageing in Modern Society*. London: Croom Helm.

Blakemore K. (1983). Ageing in the inner city – a comparison of old blacks and whites. In Jerrome D. (ed.), *Ageing in Modern Society*. London: Croom Helm.

Bond J. and Carstairs V. (1982). *Services for the Elderly*. Scottish Health Service Studies no. 42. Edinburgh: Scottish Home and Health Department.

Campbell A., Mitchell S. and Earwicker J. (1981). *The Elderly at Home in Hammersmith and Fulham*. The London Borough of Hammersmith and Fulham.

Copeland J., Kelleher M., Smith A. and Devlin P. (1986). The well, the mentally ill, the old, and the old old: a community survey of elderly persons in London. *Ageing and Society*, **6**, 417–33.

Cumming E. and Henry W. (1961). *Growing Old*. New York: Basic Books.

de Beauvoir S. (1972). *Old Age*. London: Weidenfeld and Nicholson.

DHSS (1986). *Neighbourhood Nursing – A Focus for Care*. Report of the Community Nursing Review (Chairman: Mrs Julia Cumberlege). London: HMSO.

DHSS (1987). *Promoting Better Health*. Cmnd 247. London: HMSO.

Eastman M. (1984). *Old Age Abuse*. London: Age Concern.

Elder G. (1977). *The Alienated – Growing Old Today*. Writers' and Readers' Publishing Cooperative.

Evers H. (1984). Old woman's self-perceptions of dependency and some implications for service provision. *Journal of Epidemiology and Community Health*, **38**, 306–9.

Family Policy Studies (1986). *An Ageing Population*. Fact sheet 2. Witley Press.

Goodman C. (1986). Research on the informal carer: a selected literature review. *Journal of Advanced Nursing*, **11**, 705–12.

Griffiths R. (1988). *Community Care: Agenda for Action*. London: HMSO.

Grundy E. (1987). Community care for the elderly. *British Medical Journal*, **294**, 626–9.

Hunt A. (1978). *The Elderly at Home*. London: HMSO.

Johnson M. (1986). The meaning of old age, in Redfern S. (ed.) *Nursing Elderly People*. Churchill Livingstone.

Lessing D. (1983). *The Diaries of Jane Somers*. Penguin.

Nissel M. and Bonnerjea L. (1982). *Family Care of the Handicapped Elderly: Who Pays?* London: Policy Studies Institute.

OPCS (1985). *Mid 1984 Population Estimates for England and Wales.* Reference PPI 85/1. London: OPCS.

OPCS (1986). *Labour Force Survey.* Ref. LFS86/2. London: OPCS.

Parker G. (1985). *With Due Care and Attention.* A review of research on informal care. Family Policy Studies Centre.

Snow T. (1981). *Services for Old Age: A Growing Crisis in London.* London: Age Concern.

Strang J., Craine N. and Acheson R. (1983) Team care of elderly patients in general practice. *British Medical Journal,* **286,** (6368) 851–4.

Townsend P. (1957). *The Family Life of Old People – An Enquiry in East London.* London: Routledge Kegan Paul.

Walker A. (1982). Dependency and old age. *Social Policy and Administration,* **16,** (2), 115–34.

Wheeler R. (1986). Housing policy and elderly people, in Phillipson C. and Walker A. (eds), *Ageing and Social Policy.* Gower.

Wilcocks D. (1986). Residential care, in Phillipson C. and Walker A. (eds), *Ageing and Social Policy.* Gower.

9

Conclusion

ALISON WHILE

Surroundings have long been acknowledged as influential. Indeed, the existence of open spaces and holidays in mountainous regions and beside the sea are generally viewed as tonics in our everyday existence. However, it is not entirely clear to what extent the physical environment affects the human condition and, further, whether inner city environments constitute a 'special case'.

There is considerable evidence that social and personal problems tend to concentrate within the inner areas of large cities (Brown and Madge, 1982). Indeed, in 1977 (a) The Department of the Environment calculated that about one in fourteen of the population live in extreme poverty and deprivation in inner city locations. The typical features of inner city environments have already been catalogued earlier in this book (namely, old housing stock, poor household amenities ...). Evidence was also presented demonstrating a greater preponderance of unskilled workers, unemployment and poor educational attainment. And interestingly a White Paper (Department of Environment, 1977b) contended that inner city areas seem to attract people with alcohol, drug or other personal troubles, as well as large numbers of ethnic minorities. Further, Rutter and Madge (1976) reviewed evidence that crime, delinquency and psychiatric disorders occurred to a greater extent in inner city areas than elsewhere.

The evidence seems to suggest an association between personal troubles and the inner city environment. However, the evidence does not support the thesis that inner cities throw up a unique pattern of problems, but rather there is an excess of disadvantage which varies from one location to another and, indeed, concentrations of problems and disadvantage have been found on council estates outside inner city areas (English, 1979).

Further, it is erroneous to describe people simply by where they live because it is clear that not only are there major differences between different inner city areas, but also enormous contrasts in the circumstances of different inner city residents. Townsend (1976) has argued that regardless of the definition of deprivation, there will be more deprivation missed by such areas than recognized, unless about half the area of the country is involved in the analysis. It is clear that inner city areas do not have the monopoly on deprivation and personal troubles.

However, there is undoubtedly much disadvantage in inner cities which is only in part ameliorated by greater use of personal social services (Imber, 1977). Indeed, family needs are further evidenced by more frequent reception of inner city children into care (House of Commons, 1980). But, it is dangerous to label inner city residents as different from other people, because not all households are disadvantaged in the same way. All households may indeed be exposed to the decaying environment and the stigma of such an address, but in other respects there is much variation in social handicap or disadvantage. Brown and Madge (1982) have further argued that even within families, different children are affected to varying extents. And they were able to demonstrate the invulnerability of some children despite quite substantial adversity in their lives.

THE VULNERABLE GROUPS

The research is conclusive in indicating that pre-school children are most affected by their home environment — not only are infant mortality rates higher in some inner city areas, but also the dependence of this group of the population upon their family for their well-being exposes them particularly to their family's 'troubles'. For example, low household income may trap families in substandard housing in which limited space prevents safe play and the development of normal family relationships. Indeed, these very circumstances may oblige a mother to go out to work and leave her infant with a less than ideal childminder or, alternatively, the stresses of home life may precipitate psychological ill-health in parents and affect how they react with their children. Graham (1980) has shown that parents overwhelmed in this way are at greater risk of causing a non-accidental injury to their children. A particularly worrying phenomenon in inner cities is the high proportion of single parents who do not have an intimate confiding relationship to sustain them through their troubles; the consequences of this are further exacerbated by changes in family and social networks so that professional support has become particularly important to family well-being.

School children are also sensitive to family problems and circumstance. Substandard housing and poverty are no less important to the well-being of children at school – completion of homework requires a home conducive to study and participation in school life means the wearing of wellington boots, soft shoes, football boots. ... Family disharmony has also been found to have repercussions on school behaviour, psychological distur- bance and delinquency (Rutter and Madge, 1976); indeed, levels of stress at home may have profound consequences. It seems that parents feel obliged to sacrifice the interests of their children in order to maintain reasonable relationships with their neighbours and may well impose severe restrictions upon their children's play activities (Wilson and Herbert, 1978). The nature of the physical environment further encourages parental repression with realistic fears of the danger of road traffic and child molesters, and the temptation to engage in vandalism, petty crime or deviant behaviour in vacant houses. The limited scholastic achievement of children from deprived backgrounds was discussed in Chapter 3 and it is worrying that progress is worse among poor children in the inner city than many other groups. However, the importance of the 'ethos' of a school (Rutter et al, 1979) as a contributor to pupil outcome will perhaps be explored by inner city teaching staff – the needs of teachers will, however, require addressing.

Transition from childhood to adulthood is a time of emotional upheaval, however, psycho-social difficulties which arise during this period, are unlikely to be a direct consequence of growing up in the inner city but rather a continuation of difficulties seated in early childhood. However, inner city youth faces a chronic lack of opportunities on leaving school and although unemployment cannot be held fully responsible for the riots in Brixton, Lord Scarman identified unemployment as a contributory factor. And indeed the author of Chapter 4 argues that this lack of employ- ment may encourage the adoption of deviant behaviour. Madge (1982) has also argued that the stresses of inner city life may lead young girls into early motherhood as a means of escaping a troubled home and attaining an independent income. The dismal statistics associated with school-girl motherhood were reviewed in Chapter 3 and, further, it appears that early motherhood does not provide optimal conditions for the next generation of children growing up in the inner city.

The author in Chapter 5 draws attention to the danger of labelling and so stigmatizing certain areas and their residents. It is argued that inner city residents in disadvantage deserve special help in order to overcome their adversities. The consequences of high rates of unemployment, low income, poor housing and family composition have been discussed in terms of the additional strain they place upon family life, and the evidence of Wilson and Herbert's (1978) research is quoted regarding the relative importance of environmental factors in explaining the demise of disadvantaged children in inner cities. Hillman notes the work of Madge (1983) which reviews the research identifying which children may receive less than adequate parenting; namely, those with young or immature parents, parents with institutional backgrounds, multiple problems in their family, instability of the family unit and frequent residential mobility, poor family support networks and limited personal coping mechanisms.

The evidence seems to suggest an increased incidence of mental health problems among inner city residents. However, it is not clear whether the poor environment precipates mental breakdown or whether people with mental health problems are attracted by the availability of cheap single accommodation and the unstructured social life. The authors of Chapter 7, however, argued that the stress of inner city deprivation plays its part in increasing individuals' susceptibility to breakdown. They interestingly drew attention to the vulnerability of ethnic minorities to mental health problems and dilemmas faced by immigrants in assimilating their new culture.

In the desire to promote the well-being of future generations it is all too easy to neglect the elderly in the inner cities. The author of Chapter 8 argues that old people are not a homogeneous group, but rather a collection of people with varying needs. And although living alone may not necessarily be associated with vulnerability, physical incapacity and bereavement are associated with greater risk. Very real poverty increases the demise of the elderly people in the inner cities and it is noteworthy that as many as 35% of old people do not claim their benefit entitlement. The effect of the new benefit system has yet to be evaluated,

however, it appears that some old people will lose some of their
benefit and with the exception of the community-care grant and
funeral payment, payments from the Social Fund are recoverable
by the State. Indeed, the new system has been criticized as
penalizing thrift. Chapter 8 highlights the needs of carers who
have been all too easily overlooked, and of particular relevance
to inner city professionals is the stretching of the informal caring
network with the loosening of the family ties and increased
mobility. Some, indeed, would argue that neglect of the needs of
informal carers may allow such deterioration of the family
dynamics that old-age abuse takes place.

MEETING NEEDS

It would be easy to expound how a major injection of resources
could improve the inner city environment, increase opportunities
and prevent these areas from attracting people with economic
and social problems. However, it is most unlikely that funds of
this magnitude will be made available in the current economic
climate. It is more constructive to consider how professionals can
improve their practice within current resource constraints
through sensitivity and innovation.

Chapter 2 described a number of improvements introduced to
child health services in different areas in an attempt to be more
sensitive to population needs. They included changes to a child
health clinic provision in Nottingham in order to attract an older
and more deprived pre-school child population hitherto reluctant
to avail themselves of the provision and various changes in
health visiting practice. The adoption of parent-held child health
records and their active use was also suggested as a method of
overcoming poor information transfer. The very limited provision of child care for working parents appears to be an in-
superable problem, with mothers in manual work and from ethnic
minorities being forced to accept less than satisfactory arrangements, and without increased resources it is hard to see how the
situation may be improved. However, some parents gain much
from their membership of support groups and no large increase
in resources would be required to foster the development of a
group in their everyday practice.

Chapter 3 reviewed the needs of school children and it was
apparent that good support during school life is of paramount

importance. Working parents need to be encouraged to provide for their younger children on their return from school and during school holidays and the National Out of School Alliance runs a comprehensive up-to-date directory of the various schemes available. More effective use of the health and social services will depend upon these services making themselves more understandable and acceptable to school children and their families. Indeed, the author of Chapter 5 addresses this very issue and argues that sensitive professional practice is of paramount importance if consumers are not to feel alienated. The school nursing service should be available to all school children and perhaps this provides the opportunity for a health worker to promote healthy behaviour and engage in counselling of families and children so that they maximize their opportunities. The Leeds Leaving Care Scheme and Park View House, Sheffield, provided good examples of innovations to meet the needs of particular children.

The author of Chapter 4 has tabulated provisions designed to help meet the needs of youth. It is clear that the loss of employment opportunities for young people is of great concern and has resulted in the development of a plethora of provisions in an attempt to facilitate the absorption of school-leavers into the job market. The adoption of deviant behaviour in the wake of unemployment and limited opportunity has received recent media attention and provisions have been developed to assist young people with drug-abuse problems — there are many excellent examples of local initiatives to help the abusers and their families. Homelessness is also apparently increasing among young people and Centrepoint, the Soho project, and Alone in London are examples of specific provisions developed to meet the needs of a particular section of youth.

An important source of help to many individuals and families is the general practitioner service. Chapter 6 has discussed in detail the various problems facing the service and how these problems may be overcome. However, only time will tell whether the recommendations of the White Paper (DHSS, 1987) will be implemented and, in the meantime, it will depend upon the general practitioners themselves as to whether they improve the service they offer.

No single model of inner city psychiatric services exists, rather, different areas have developed different approaches to meet the needs of their populations. Chapter 7 emphasized that most peoply rely upon general practice services for care, with only a minority of people receiving specialist psychiatric help. The authors discussed the contribution of different mental health professionals in some detail and described examples of community-care service models which have been developed as an alternative to hospital care. However, it is clear that improvements could be made to improve the support given to mental illness patients and their family and friends. A contribution to improved services for the mentally ill may be a further extension of community psychiatric nursing services, social work and psychologist support, so that they may be able to work effectively within the primary care setting, along with other interested professionals, so maintaining patients in their own homes and thus avoiding hospital admission as much as possible.

Lack of sensitivity in the support provisions for elderly people from ethnic minorities was highlighted in Chapter 8 and indeed the author outlined how professionals may enhance or reduce dependence of old people through their attitudes and practice. Evers' (1984) work emphasizes the need for professionals to identify how individual old people perceive their dependence so that they may offer appropriate support. A number of interesting initiatives were described in Chapter 8 and provide examples of how the needs of old people and their carers may be met.

GROUNDS FOR OPTIMISM?

While clearly a large increase in resources to our inner city areas would markedly reduce the deprivation and social disadvantage of the residents, the reality is that such an injection of funds is unlikely in the foreseeable future. However, it has been demonstrated by the contributors to this book that changes and improvements in professional practice can contribute significantly to the support and life experience of the residents. Thus there are indeed grounds for optimism – not for overwhelming changes in the circumstances of inner city residents, but for changes in professional practice which make it more sensitive to the needs of the consumers. There is also increasing evidence that individuals are able to overcome overwhelming adversities in their lives and gain strength from these experiences, or at least emerge relatively unscathed. Underlying the ability to survive adversities is the experience of good family relationships

(Madge, 1982) and perhaps this gives a pointer as to where support resources should be focused. Elder (1979) found, for instance, that boys are less resilient to adversity if there is family discord and Madge (1982) found that families are more able to successfully endure the consequences of paternal unemployment where the marital relationship is good. Indeed, Madge argues that levels of stress reported by inner city families are a reflection of their home atmosphere; that is, whether they feel the atmosphere is 'happy', 'intermediate' or 'unhappy'.

REFERENCES

Brown M. and Madge N. (1982). *Despite the Welfare State*. London: Heinemann Educational.

Department of Environment (1977a). *Housing Policy: A Consultative Document*. Cmnd 6851. London: HMSO.

Department of Environment (1977b). *A Policy for the Inner Cities*. Cmnd 6845. London: HMSO.

Department of Health and Social Security (1987). *Promoting Better Health*. Cm 249. London: HMSO.

Elder G. H. Jr (1979). Historical change in life patterns and personality, in Baltes P. B. and Brim O. G. Jr.(eds): *Life-Span Development and Behavior*, Vol 2. London: Academic Press.

English J. (1979). Access and deprivation in local authority housing, in Jones C. (ed.): *Urban Deprivation and the Inner City*. London: Croom Helm.

Evers H. (1984). Old woman's self-perceptions of dependency and some implications for service provision. *Journal of Epidemiology and Community Health*, **38**, 306–9.

Graham H. (1980). Mothers' accounts of anger and aggression towards their babies, in Frude N. (ed.): *Psychological Approaches to Child Abuse*. London: Batsford.

House of Commons (1980). *Children in Care in England and Wales*. March 1978. London: HMSO.

Imber V. (1977). *A Classification of the English Personal Social Service Authorities*. DHSS Statistical and Research Report Series, No. 16, London: HMSO.

Madge N. J. H. (1982). Growing up in the Inner City. *Journal of Royal Society of Health*, **102** (6), 261–5.

Madge N. (ed.) (1983). *Families at Risk*. London: Heinemann Educational.

Rutter M. and Madge N. (1976). *Cycles of Disadvantage*. London: Heinemann Educational.

Rutter M., Maughan B., Mortimer P. and Ouston J. (1979). *Fifteen Thousand Hours: Secondary Schools and their Effects upon Children*. London: Open Books.
Townsend P. (1976). Area deprivation policies. *New Statesman*. 6 Aug.
Wilson H. and Herbert G. W. (1978). *Parents and Children in the Inner City*. London: Routledge & Kegan Paul.

Index